The Brain

The Brain:

Mystery of Matter and Mind

U.S.NEWS BOOKS Washington, D. C.

U.S.NEWS BOOKS

THE HUMAN BODY
The Brain:
Mystery of Matter and Mind

Editor/Publisher
Roy B. Pinchot

Series Editor
Judith Gersten

Contributing Editor
Linda S. Glisson

Book Design
David M. Seager

Art Direction
The Glusker Group, Inc.

Cover Design
Moonink Communications

Staff Writers
Wayne Barrett
Kathy E. Goldberg
Karen Jensen
Edward O. Welles, Jr.
Anthony S. Pitch

Director of Text Research
William Rust

Text Researchers
Susana Barañano
Heléne Goldberg
Bruce A. Lewenstein
Barbara L. Lewis

Picture Editor
Leah Bendavid-Val

Picture Researchers
Gregory Johnson
Leora Kahn
David Ross
Jean Shapiro
Johanna Boublik

Director of Production
Harold F. Chevalier

Production Coordinator
Diane Breunig Freed

Copy Staff
Carol Bashara
Ina Bloomberg
Barbara M. Clark
Raymond Ferry
Sharon Turner

Quality Control Director
Joseph Postilion

Director of Sales
James Brady

Business Planning
Robert Licht

Fulfillment Director
Debra Hasday Fanshel

Cover Art
Paul Giovanopoulos

Author

Jack Fincher is the author of *Lefties*, a study of left-handedness, and *Human Intelligence*, which received an award from the American Medical Writers Association. A former bureau chief for *Life* magazine, Mr. Fincher has recently written for *Smithsonian, Reader's Digest* and *People* magazines.

Series Consultants

Donald M. Engelman, Molecular Biophysicist and Biochemist at Yale University, is a Guest Biophysicist at the Brookhaven National Laboratory in New York. A specialist in biological structure, Dr. Engelman has published research in American and European journals. From 1976 to 1980, he was chairman of the Molecular Biology Study Section at the National Institutes of Health.

Stanley Joel Reiser is Associate Professor of Medical History at Harvard Medical School and codirector of the Kennedy Interfaculty Program in Medical Ethics at the University. He is the author of *Medicine and the Reign of Technology* and coeditor of *Ethics in Medicine: Historical Perspectives and Contemporary Concerns.*

Harold C. Slavkin, Professor of Biochemistry at UCLA, directs the Graduate Program in Craniofacial Biology and also serves as Chief of the Laboratory for Developmental Biology in the University's Gerontology Center. His research on the genetic basis of congenital defects of the head and neck has been widely published.

Lewis Thomas is Chancellor of the Memorial Sloan-Kettering Cancer Center in New York City. A member of the National Academy of Sciences, Dr. Thomas has served on advisory councils of the National Institutes of Health. He has written *The Medusa and the Snail* and *The Lives of a Cell*, which received the 1974 National Book Award in Arts and Letters.

Consultants *for* The Brain

Jack M. Fein is Assistant Professor of Vascular Surgery at the Albert Einstein College of Medicine in New York. He practices neurosurgery at Albert Einstein College Hospital and at two other New York City hospitals. Recipient of the Irving Wright Award for Research in Cerebrovascular Diseases, Dr. Fein is coauthor of a book on microsurgical techniques and is preparing a four-volume series on cerebrovascular surgery.

Charles J. Furst is Associate Research Psychologist at the UCLA Neuropsychiatric Institute. He taught psychology at Dartmouth College and at California State University. Dr. Furst also served as consultant to the National Institute on Alcohol Abuse and Alcoholism. His book *Origins of the Mind* examines the physiological basis of consciousness.

Solomon H. Snyder is Director of the Department of Neuroscience and Professor of Neuroscience, Pharmacology and Psychiatry at Johns Hopkins University. He received the 1978 Albert Lasker Medical Research Award in Basic Biomedical Research for his discovery of opiate receptors in the brain. Dr. Snyder has also written five books on the brain and behavior.

Seymour Diamond is Adjunct Associate Professor of Neurology at the Chicago Medical School. Recently elected Executive Officer, Migraine and Headache Research Group for the World Federation of Neurology, he also serves as Executive Director of the American Association for the Study of Headache and the National Migraine Foundation.

Picture Consultants

Amram Cohen is General Surgery Resident at the Walter Reed Army Medical Center in Washington, D.C.

Richard G. Kessel, Professor of Zoology at the University of Iowa, studies cells, tissues and organs with scanning and transmission electron microscopy instruments. He is coauthor of two books on electron microscopy.

Illustrators

Louis Bory, Tracy Garner, Edward Allgor, George Kelvin, Adolph Brotman, Ilil Arbel, Walter Rane, Esperance Shatara, Mel Keefer, Katrina Taylor, Joseph Papin, Andy Christie, Leonard Dank/*Medical Illustrations Co.*, Jim Ruttencutter

---

**Library of Congress
Cataloging in Publication Data**

Fincher, Jack, 1930 –
   The brain, mystery of matter and mind.

   (The Human body)
   Includes index.
   1. Brain. I. Title. II. Series: Human body.
QP376.F48   612'.82   81–3052
                           AACR2

ISBN 0–89193–601–7
ISBN 0–89193–631–9 (leatherbound)
ISBN 0–89193–661–0 (lib. bdg.)

20 19 18 17 16 15 14 13 12 11
10   9   8   7   6   5   4   3   2   1

Contents

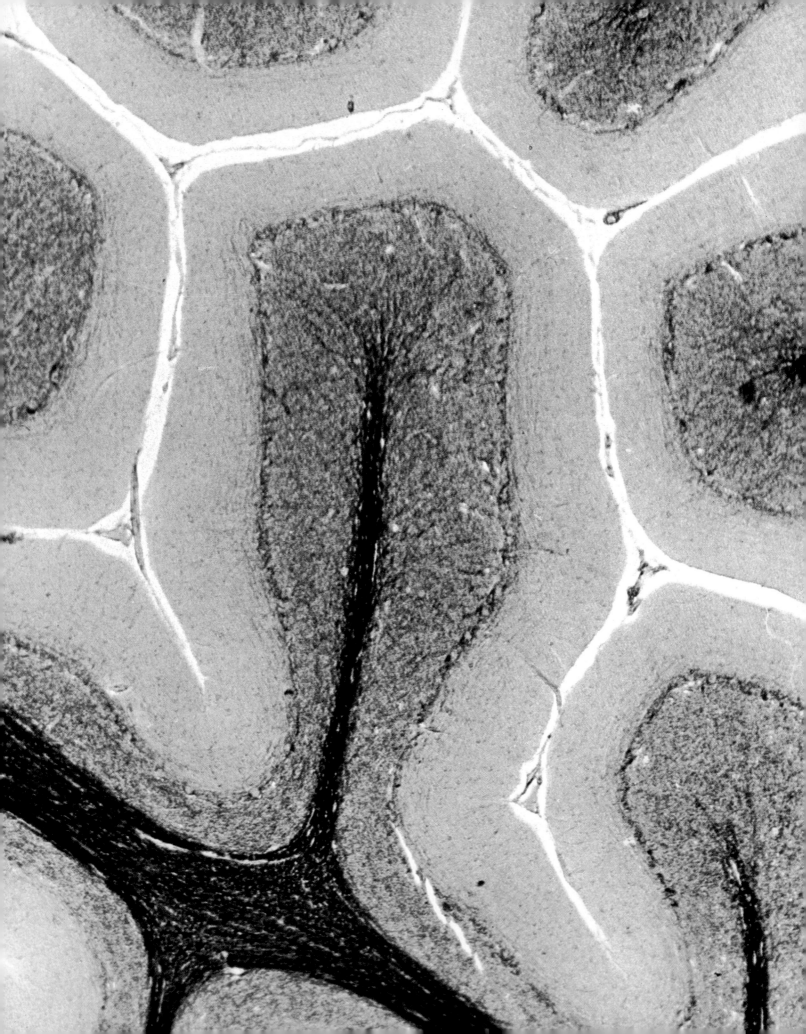

Introduction:

The Enchanted Loom

Parquet patterns of the cerebellum, greatly magnified, reveal the intricate construction of the brain. Dark nerve filaments fringe the cortex and fade into yellow-stained core matter, pathways for impulses to regulate body movements.

Every cell of the human body is ruled by the brain. Its commanding presence orders sensation, movement, thought, a lifetime of memory and dream. What makes this so is the central nervous system, a maze of nerve fibers linking all areas of the body to cells in the fabric of the brain. Within that "enchanted loom," romanticized physiologist Sir Charles Sherrington, "millions of flashing shuttles weave a dissolving pattern, always a meaningful pattern, though never an abiding one."

Object of mystery and superstition through most of history, mankind's brain has revealed itself only in recent centuries. Ancient Greeks reasoned that thought was "the soul's walk abroad." Thinking about the brain, seeking ways to unravel its infinite mysteries, inspired the minds of great men — St. Augustine, Leonardo da Vinci, Descartes, Freud.

Anthropologist Loren Eiseley noted that both gorilla and human have "appealingly similar" brains at birth. But the human's triples in size the first year, growing "unlike anything else we know in the animal world." Problem solving, language, creating works of art — all bear witness to humankind's unique birthright.

Seeds of thought lie in furrows of dark tissue that cover the brain like a layer of fertile topsoil. From here stem conscious acts, speaking one's mind — and changing it. Within the brain's lobes echo sounds, awakening imaginations. Impulses of sight, rocketing through these spaces, stir memories. Deeper in the brain's core are rooted the origins of feelings, our pleasures and sorrows. Among the emotions twine tendrils of smell, sensing nostalgia's past.

We may see, through the eyes of science, ever more of the enchanted loom. To unveil what is known about the brain — and what is not — is to stretch the limits of imagination. Future discoveries will propel man to new thresholds of awe.

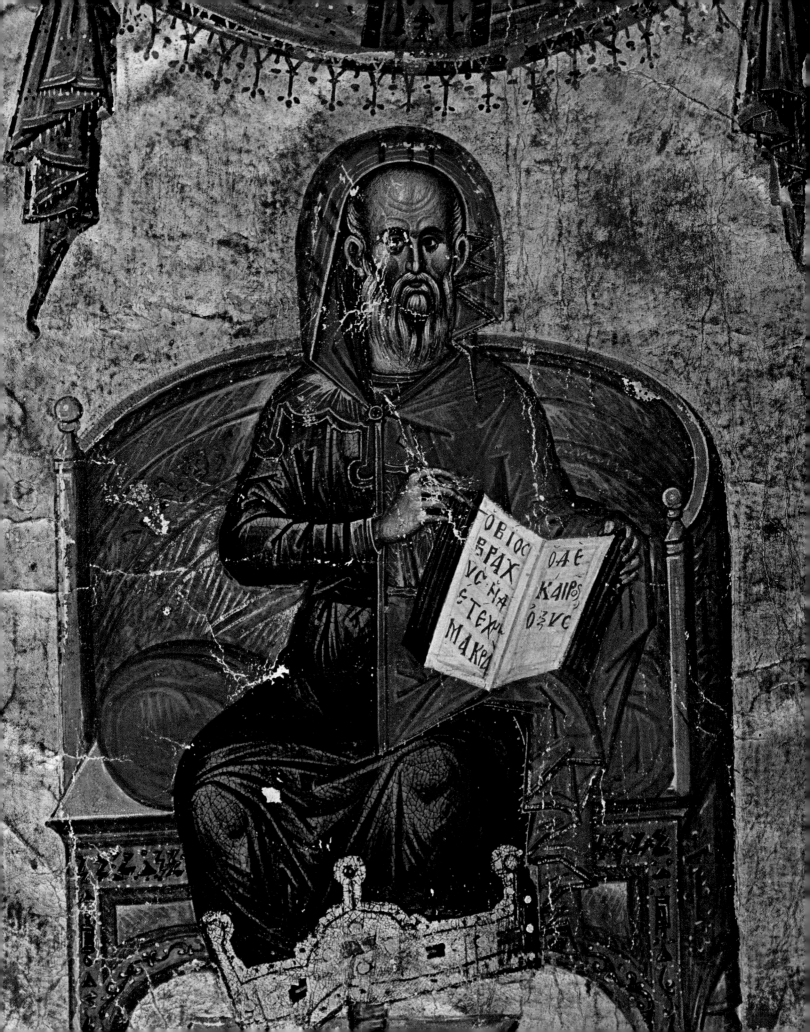

Chapter 1

The Divinest Part

What is the brain? Twenty-five centuries ago, Hippocrates, legendary father of medicine, framed an enduring answer. "Not only our pleasure, our joy and our laughter but also our sorrow, pain, grief and tears arise from the brain, and the brain alone," he declared. "With it we think and understand, see and hear, and we discriminate between the ugly and the beautiful, between what is pleasant and what is unpleasant and between good and evil."

The notion that the brain served as the organ of the mind and as the temple of the soul was not new. In the sixth century B.C., Greek philosophers Pythagoras and Alcmaeon had suggested as much. From these two thinkers Plato, a contemporary of Hippocrates, drew inspiration. Within the head's "spherical body," he rhapsodized, "is the divinest part of us and lord over all the rest."

Not so, thought Aristotle, student of Plato. Agreeing with earlier beliefs held by Hebrews, Hindus and Chinese, he championed the heart as the source of intelligence. He also deemed it the body's nerve center. The brain, Aristotle reasoned, cooled hot blood coursing up from the heart. The debate, unceasing through the centuries, moved Shakespeare to ask:

> Tell me where is fancie bred,
> Or in the heart or in the head . . .

Plato perceived the soul to be immortal, moving from body to body, and vulnerable to angry gods, who inflicted insanity, hysteria and epilepsy, the "sacred disease." Hippocrates believed the sacred disease was "nowise more divine" than others "but has a natural cause from which it originates." He asserted that "the brain is the cause of this affection" and warned against treatment by spells, amulets and "other illiberal practices." One such remedy directed the patient to "take a nail of a wrecked ship, make it into a bracelet and set therein the bone of a stag's heart

To Hippocrates, father of medicine, thought and emotion originated in the brain — not in the heart, as others believed. Portrayed here in Byzantine trappings, the ancient Greek physician opens his book to a favorite aphorism: "Life is short, and the art is long." The collected Hippocratic writings include works by many authors.

Body fluids of antiquity, called humors, also served medieval notions of health and disposition. Clockwise, melancholy patient suffers from excess of black bile; blood empassions sanguine lutist to play; a maiden, dominated by phlegm, is slow to respond to her lover; choler, too much yellow bile, makes an angry master. Today, we still speak of good and bad humors to describe temperament and mood. The four humors themselves survive as well. Melancholy is synonymous with sad and phlegmatic with un-emotional. We use sanguine to mean a ruddy or cheerful person, and choleric to describe an irritable one.

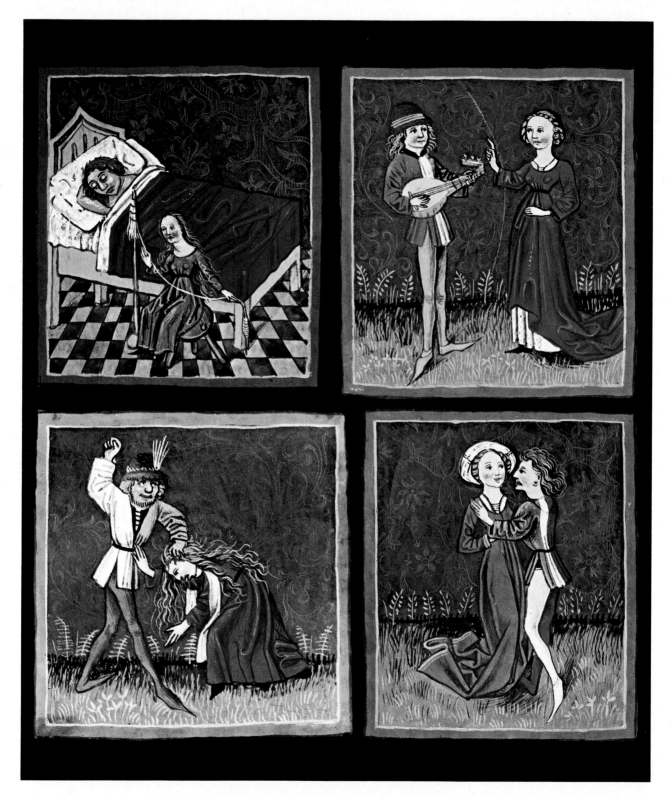

Tiny blood vessels, the rete mirabile, *web the brain in an arterial system by anatomist Vesalius. He knew the rete did not exist in humans, but included it "to agree with Galen's description."*

taken from its body whilst alive." Wear it on the left arm, the epileptic was instructed, and "you will be astonished at the result."

Hippocrates thought the brain was "the primary seat of sense," as well as a supreme gland that secreted soothing phlegm called *pituita*. From that term derived modern anatomy's pituitary gland, a tiny pendant of tissue suspended in the brain. The body's master gland, it secretes hormones that control growth and well-being. Ancient physicians, ignorant of hormones, invented humors, bodily fluids, to explain mysteries of mind and body. Phlegm, blood, yellow bile known as choler and the black bile of melancholy all interacted to cause disease or preserve health. The four humors formed a system of medicine born of logic and practiced by followers of Plato. Another system centered on the air, or *pneuma*. From the lungs, pneuma mixed with blood in the heart, then dispersed through the body. "Changed by the state of the air," the brain, Hippocrates theorized, thus gained the power of understanding.

Medieval Spirits

From philosopher and physician, from priest and pagan, a distillation of dogmas evolved governing for centuries man's perception of self. The life force, it was believed, flowed from ethereal spirits made in the body. The liver, fed by the intestines, produced natural spirit that streamed to the heart, where it was refined into vital spirit. This enriched mixture became animal spirit after it pulsed to the brain and mixed with the pneuma. Medieval physicians believed the blending took place in the *rete mirabile*, the "marvelous net" of blood vessels seen in hoofed mammals and assumed to be in the base of the human brain.

After the animal spirit was processed in the fancied rete, it supposedly trickled into the ventricles, the brain's system of cavities, for distribution through the nervous system, thought to consist of tiny tubes. Medieval sketches showed the ventricles arranged in the skull like tennis balls, a cluster of psychic cells charged with powers of *memorativa, imaginativa, cogitatia* and *sensus communis*. The shapes were drawn with artistic license from a description by Galen, the second-century Greek physician "known to the foremost

ARTERIA MAGNA, AOPTH, הנכוב HAORTI EX SI- NISTRO CORDIS SINV ORIENS, ET VITALEM SPIRITVM TOTI CORPORI DEFERENS, NATV. RALEMQVE CALOREM PER CONTRACTIONEM ET DILATATIONEM TEMPERANS.

NOTATV DIGNAE ARTERIAE MAGNAE SOBOLES CENTVM ET QVADRAGINTA SEPTEM APPARENT

11

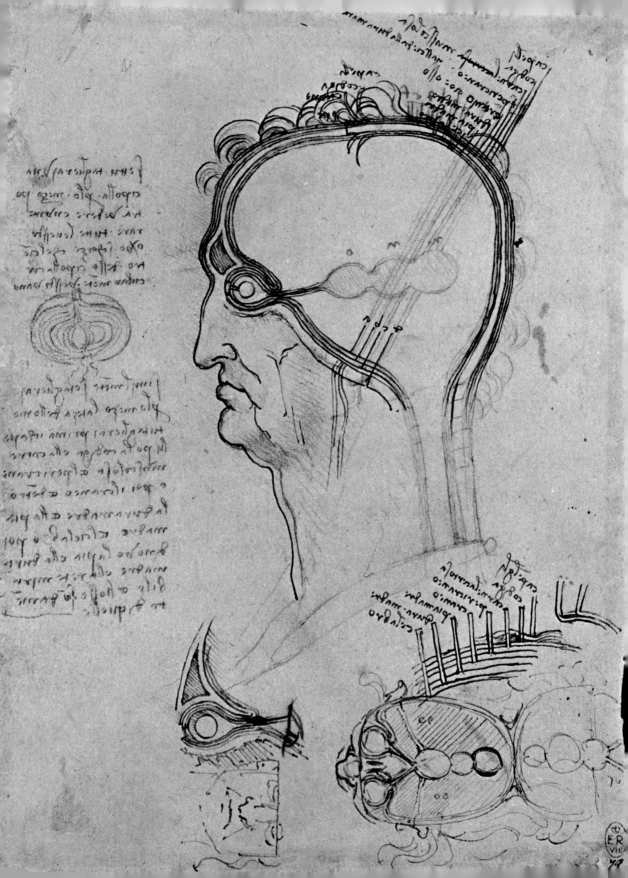

men in Rome and to all the emperors." Imagine
the branchings removed from the ventricles, he
wrote, and "what you have left is perfectly
spherical." He dissected oxen and Barbary apes
but apparently not humans in his study of anatomy, setting down his conclusions in hundreds
of treatises. Galen theorized that the "power of
sensation and of movement flows from the
brain" and that "what is rational in the soul has
its existence there." He placed the mental powers
in the marrowlike substance of the brain known
as white matter. But fourth-century theologians
Nemesius and St. Augustine favored the psychic-
cell complex, endowing the ventricles with the
soul as well as common sense.

Galen's ideas prevailed for fifteen hundred
years, forming a reservoir of medicine mixed
with myth and magic. The church and the
mosque freely borrowed from Galen, often
through Jewish physicians who, during the Dark
Ages, served as guardians of medical knowledge.
Galen's thought survives in the *Arabian Nights*,
with the caliph pondering where in the body
dwelled understanding. A slave girl's answer re-
flected Greek influence: "Allah casteth it in the
heart whence its illustrious beams ascend to the
brain and there become fixed." Such ideas, nour-
ished by time and tradition, died slowly.

Of Heretics and Kings

Heralding the Renaissance, Leonardo da Vinci,
exhilarated by his anatomical findings, declared
"I wish to work miracles." At first he copied
Galen by portraying the system of ventricles in
the approved classical manner, as spheres. The
sphere he labeled common sense was the judge of
"things offered to it by the other senses," the
place where the "soul seems to reside." That observation, evocative of St. Augustine, was neither
original nor scientific, although Leonardo boast-
ed he had dissected ten human bodies. Yet it was
an ox on which he came closest to working a
miracle. Borrowing the sculptor's device of cast-
ing bronze statues from wax forms, he poured
hot wax into an ox's ventricles, allowed it to
harden, then stripped away the flesh to reveal
the true shape of the cavities. Five centuries later,
X-rays would capture the ventricles on film.

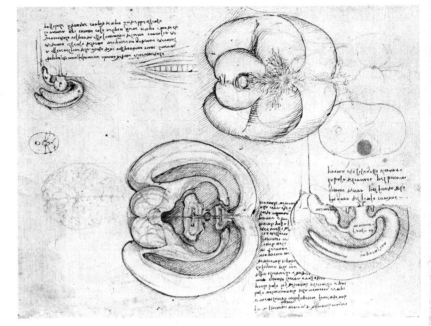

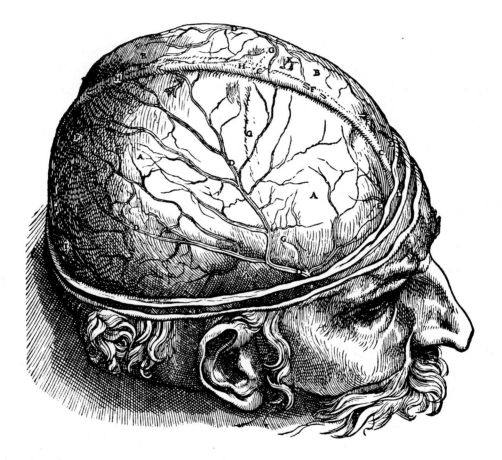

Anatomist Andreas Vesalius further weakened the ties to the ancients in 1543 with the publication of *De Humani Corporis Fabrica*, the Structure of the Human Body. The author, not yet turned thirty, employed artists from the studio of Titian — and perhaps the master himself — to reveal man's naked self as none before had dared. From the heads of executed criminals he illustrated the brain, producing drawings that revolutionized neuroanatomy. In *Fabrica* he refuted the medieval notion that the four ventricles stored separate mental faculties of imagination, judgment, cogitation and memory. Clashing with tradition, he denied the existence of the rete mirabile in humans and intimated "that very tenuous" animal spirit played no role in thinking.

Vesalius risked being branded a heretic for flouting "that crowd of philosophers and . . . theologians . . . who . . . fabricate some sort of brain from their dreams." Little did he dream

that twenty years later he would confront such a crowd at the bedside of a delirious, dying prince.

"In hasty following of a wench," Don Carlos, heir to the Spanish throne, "fell down a pair of stairs [and] broke his head." Royal physicians plastered the wound with powdered iris, birthwort and egg yolk. A Moorish quacksalver burned him with ointments. Three thousand flagellants parading outside the palace scourged themselves with whips. None of these measures succeeded in reviving Don Carlos; nor did the cold corpse of the Blessed Diego of Alcalá, brought in one night to keep vigil beside the feverish prince. Vesalius was summoned by King Philip. With hope ebbing, court physicians carried out Vesalius's instruction that the swollen eye sockets be incised and drained. Immediately the fever broke. In a few weeks the prince felt strong enough to attend a bullfight. Credit for his miraculous recovery was paid to the local relic,

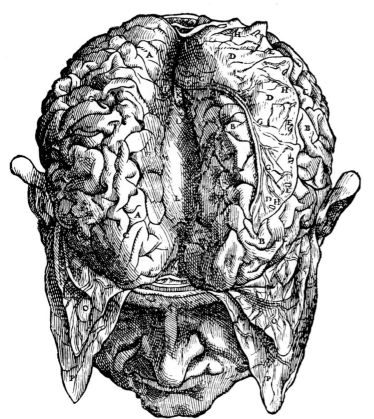

Illustrations from Vesalius's Fabrica, *said to have "established with startling suddenness the beginning of modern observational sciences and research," starkly revealed the human brain. In profile, opposite, he drew the veined dura membrane that sheathes the brain. The membrane has been cut away, above, to expose the corpus callosum between fissured hemispheres. Beseeching executioners for decapitated criminals, the anatomist often dissected brains still warm.*

Diego. Vesalius journeyed to the Holy Land — fleeing the Inquisition, some claimed.

Seventeenth-century thinkers moved in bold, new directions, but the patient did not immediately take a turn for the better. Doctors still bled him until he lost consciousness. Or they compounded folk remedies such as powdered mistletoe for the falling sickness, epilepsy, to be taken "early in the morning, in black cherry water, for some days near the full moon." Not even kings were exempt. Charles II, attended by thirteen physicians, was bled, purged, cupped and scarified. His head was shaved and blistered, and cauterizing irons branded his convulsing body. The Merry Monarch, as he was called, might well have welcomed the stroke that killed him.

Descartes's Earthen Machine

While medical treatment plodded, burdened by harmful methods and worthless brews, medical science bounded forward. The ancient Greeks had taught that "what escapes the sight of the eyes can be seized with the sight of the mind." With the development of the microscope in the seventeenth century, the eye would see for the first time how false the mind's imagery could be. Dutch cloth merchant Anton van Leeuwenhoek ground lenses of remarkable clarity in his spare time. Through them, he detected "very little animalcules" — protozoa and bacteria — as well as blood corpuscles. He also saw that nerve tissue "consisted of diverse, very small threads or vessels lying by one another." He wondered if "these vessels might not be those that conveyed the animal spirits through the spinal marrow."

At nearly the same time Oxford professor Thomas Willis described his "doctrine of the nerves." In *Cerebri Anatome*, illustrated by Sir Christopher Wren, Willis reclassified the cranial nerves, naming nine pairs, and traced the flow of blood to the brain. He accurately concluded that thought arose from the cerebrum, the looming hemispheres of the brain.

Willis was one among equals in a century celebrated for its brilliant minds. The poetic genius of Shakespeare gave to Falstaff the explanation for the apoplexy suffered by Henry IV: "a kind of sleeping in the blood, a whoreson tingling. . . .

15

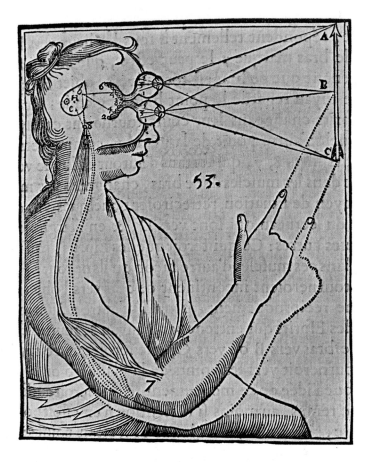

Distorted for simplicity, this enigmatic figure displays with pointing finger the mechanical nature of the nervous system, as envisioned by seventeenth-century philosopher René Descartes. Light transmits images to the retinas, stimulating animal spirit to activate the teardrop pineal gland. It then energizes nerves in the arm to produce movement. Fearful of the charge of heresy, Descartes did not publish the Treatise of Man, from which this sketch is taken. He intended the Treatise as part of a larger work explaining all of nature and man's place in it. Published in 1664, fourteen years after his death, it encompassed what are now many disciplines of science.

It hath its original from much grief, from study and perturbation of the brain. I have read the cause of its effects in Galen." Many, including the proud Fellows of the Royal Society, had read Galen. William Harvey, physician to lords and kings, observed that bodily sensations traveled through sensory nerves to the brain, and that motor nerves directed the muscles of the body. Marcello Malpighi, anatomist at Pisa, trained his microscopes on the cerebral cortex — the blanket of tissue that enfolds the brain's core — and saw a dark maze of minute cells. Here, the elusive animal spirit must be secreted, theorized Leyden professor Franz de le Boë. Rechristening himself Sylvius, a fraternal gesture to the ancients, he left that name on the deep lateral groove of the cortex: the fissure of Sylvius.

The cerebral cortex began to be viewed as more than a protective covering for the brain. Paradoxically, before men thought to ask if it served a higher function, part of the answer had been recorded: ". . . it is to be conceived that the motor force, or the nerves themselves, take their origin from the brain, where the fantasy is located." That declaration from René Descartes would find confirmation in the work of later investigators. Pinpointing the brain's components for specific functions was not a major concern of Descartes, although he knew of Galen's work and had studied the anatomy of cattle at slaughterhouses.

A towering figure in this age of scientific revolution, Descartes "resolved to take myself as an object of study and to employ all the powers of my mind in choosing the paths I should follow." The paths he chose contributed to the founding of modern psychology. Following in his wake, philosopher Arthur Schopenhauer observed that Descartes "placed . . . reason on its own feet by teaching men to use their own brains, in the place of which the Bible had previously served on the one hand, and Aristotle on the other."

Descartes invented a model man in which the body was "but a statue, an earthen machine," with the nerves likened to the plumbing of fountains adorning royal gardens. He compared the pulsing water to the driving force of animal spirit, "of which the heart is the source and the brain's cavities the water main." Breathing and other involuntary actions were automatic, like a mill wheel turning from the water's continuous flow. Such a model might be applied to all living creatures. Descartes said that "when there shall be a rational soul in this machine, it will have its chief seat in the brain and will there reside like the turncock." Twist the valve and, "through the intervention of the nerves, the soul will have different feelings." Thus did God, "a substance infinite," join body and soul. Descartes selected the tiny pineal gland nestled deep in the brain as the physical abode of the soul, for he thought it a vital organ to the brain's blood supply.

Flawed but profound, Descartes's image of the body and soul furnished grist for thinkers to come. How, they would wonder, did the mind comprehend the existence of the matter it inhabited? How could one mind be sure it was not alone and all else a delusion? Descartes himself believed this was a matter best understood by not thinking too much about it.

Mining the Cortex

But thought, snapping the bonds of church and tradition, dashed headlong into the eighteenth century, eager to examine the mysteries of mesmerism, the magic of magnetism and the pseudoscience of phrenology. Dawning too was the science of electrophysiology, exorcising at last the spell of psychic spirits. There was something even for the patient, a calibrated contraption called the thermometer.

Franz Anton Mesmer, friend of Mozart, developed techniques using so-called animal magnetism. His patients clasped hands around a pool bristling with magnetized iron bars as Mesmer led them into trances — "mesmerizing" them. Although Paris society hailed him, a commission of the *Académie des Sciences*, which included ambassador Benjamin Franklin, soberly concluded that something "having no existence can consequently have no use." The convulsive symptoms observed in participants were "ascribed to the imagination called into action." But neither the commission nor Mesmer understood the force that hypnotic suggestion exerted on the imagination, a discovery that Sigmund Freud and other framers of modern psychiatry would exploit.

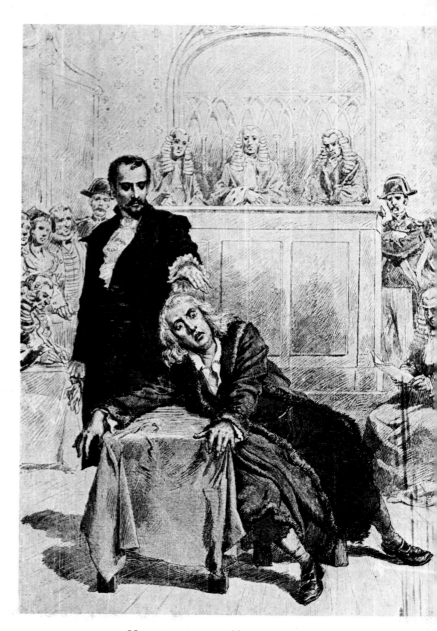

Hypnotic trance yields a courtroom confession in this period print. The practice grew out of Franz Anton Mesmer's seances in Paris employing "animal magnetism" — actually the power of suggestion. Mesmer, one writer concluded, "had rediscovered the power of the medicine man."

Reading skulls for clues to human character titillated Europe for half a century. This ersatz science of phrenology, introduced in the 1790s by Franz Joseph Gall, stemmed from his perception that people with

bulging eyes had good memories. "Why," he wondered, "should not the other faculties also have their visible external characteristics?" Mapped skulls, like the one below, marked the birth of a fad.

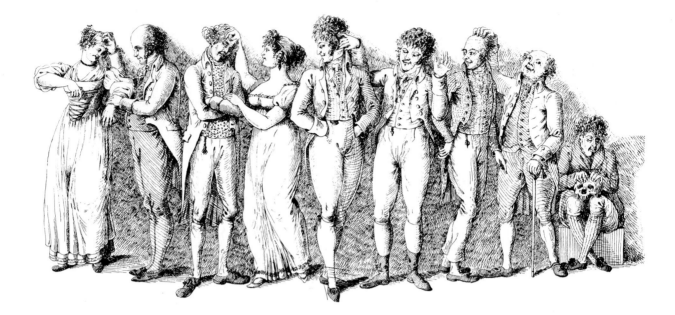

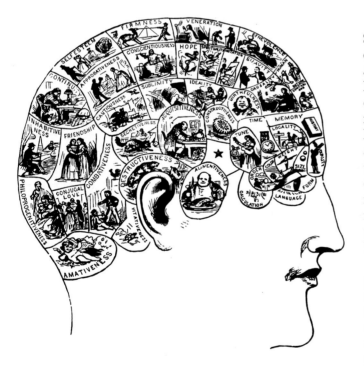

Between the time of Descartes and Mesmer, Swedish professor Emanuel Swedenborg experienced visions of heaven and hell. Before turning away from science, which he feared was leading him toward a godless, mechanistic interpretation of the mind, Swedenborg made several determinations of brain function that were far ahead of his time. His observations, not published until almost a century and a half after they were written, located and defined the motor cortex, the ear-to-ear band of gray matter where voluntary motion is triggered. He theorized that "when the mind is heated with passion . . . the lungs likewise boil up," correctly linking respiration to brain activity instead of heartbeat.

The cortex proved to be a rich area for Europe's powdered and wigged prospectors. They staked out cranial claims, rigged electrical probes and opened skulls with drills and blades. Neapolitan anatomist Domenico Cotugno discovered that shock-absorbing cerebrospinal fluid, not animal spirit, filled the ventricles. Marie Antoinette's physician, Felix Vicq d'Azyr, hardened a brain in alcohol and observed that the rawhide-thick cortex consisted of several layers. About the same time, Swiss professor Albrecht von Haller traced the relationship of nerves from the limbs to the

Lace-collared phrenologist measures cranial bumps of a gullible client, object of ridicule for nineteenth-century satirists. Gall's followers subdivided the head into more than a hundred areas as "newly discov-

ered organs" were added. Despite its far-fetched claims, phrenology served to stimulate interest in the cerebral cortex. Instead of feeling for bumps, scientists probed the cortex to localize motor functions.

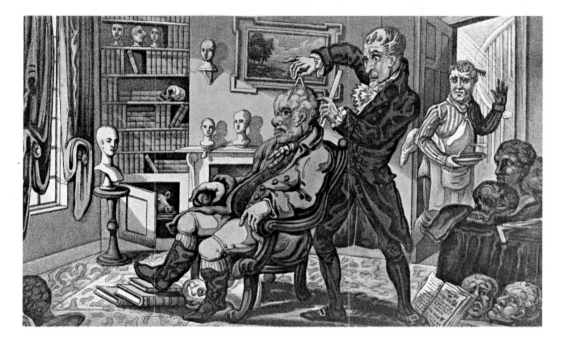

cortex. He believed the nerves transmitted sensibility through a "very thin and invisible fluid."

Electrical stimulation of the cortex preoccupied scientists, among them naturalist Felice Fontana, who attached probes to the heads of decapitated criminals. His contemporary, anatomist Luigi Galvani, demonstrated with frogs that an electrical charge caused muscles to contract. Such experiments spurred efforts to prove the existence of animal electricity, a new theory designed to displace timeworn animal spirit and nerve fluid as messengers of the mind. But the eighteenth century and the next would run their course before electrical pulses of the brain could be detected and measured by such devices as psychiatrist Hans Berger's electroencephalograph.

Mind and Matter

Near the turn of the nineteenth century, phrenology made its debut. The pseudoscience created by flamboyant Franz Joseph Gall lured thousands to skull-adorned salons to have their heads read. Phrenologists examined cranial bumps and depressions to locate underlying mental faculties, determining in the process subtle differences that purportedly indicated too much or too little of various personality traits. Holy Roman Emperor

Francis II refused to grant publication of Gall's doctrine in Vienna lest "some lose their heads over it." Gall found the freedom to pursue his practice in Napoleon's Paris, and published drawings of more than two dozen cranial areas he defined as organs.

Gall's guesswork was not without scientific value. He had introduced the idea of localizing mental functions in the cerebral cortex, a task that others would later perform with precision. But it was as an anatomist that he excelled. Said surgeon Pierre Flourens, whose own knife would soon expose phrenology's errors, "I shall never forget the feeling I experienced the first time I saw Gall dissect a brain. It seemed to me that I had never seen this organ before." Gall demonstrated remarkable insight by assigning mental powers to the cortex. But he went too far when he pretended to assess a person's character by the shape of the head.

His downfall came when Flourens, deciding to test theories of phrenology, sliced away living tissue of animal brains. Where Gall's touch had divined the seat of amorousness, Flourens's excision resulted in the loss of integrated movement. Where Gall's fingers forecast higher faculties, Flourens's scalpel numbed the senses, crippling

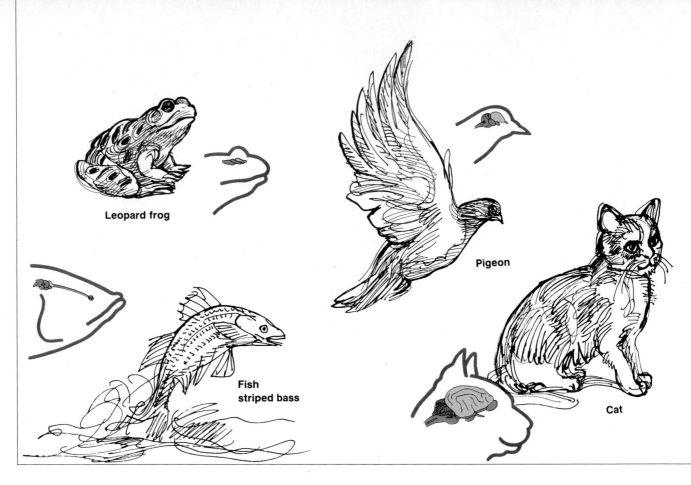

Leopard frog

Pigeon

**Fish
striped bass**

Cat

voluntary action. Although he sometimes cut across different functional areas with ambiguous results, Flourens demonstrated conclusively that matter and mind were interrelated.

Flourens mirrored the vitality of French medicine after the Revolution. Chemist Louis Pasteur sounded the tone of the times: "In the field of observation, chance only favors prepared minds." No mind was better prepared than that of Claude Bernard. Pasteur saw him not as a physiologist but as physiology itself. Bernard devised new vivisectional techniques and postulated how the *milieu intérieur*, the body's internal environment, reacted to external influences. "A strong nerve stimulus," his biography states, "such as may be provoked by terror or deep emotion, will stop the heart long enough to prevent the arrival of blood in the brain, and the result will be fainting. A milder stimulus will stop the heart more briefly . . . but the function will be resumed with an increase in the tempo, fluttering, or palpitation, which will send more blood to the brain, and result in a blush." Here recast in a scientific mold was the ancient belief that blood from the heart tempered the brain. Here was the ghost of Aristotle whispering through the centuries, "I told you so."

Bernard's idea that body fluids could affect emotional behavior echoed the humoral theory of the ancients. His contemporary, Charles Edouard Brown-Séquard, taught that the body's adrenals and other glands produced the vital secretions now known as hormones. He confirmed, author Harley Williams wrote, "that we move our limbs, live our emotions, and think our thoughts through a complex but very beautiful mechanism that lies between nerve tendrils so fine as to be invisible, and fluid secretions that are powerful yet beyond the reach of chemistry."

From the middle of the 1800s other questing Frenchmen significantly lengthened their reach. Jean Charcot, clinician, artist, mentor of Freud, first demonstrated in humans how brain damage to the cortex's motor centers produced paralysis and epilepsy. Pierre Paul Broca, great anatomist of the brain, discovered the area in the left cerebral hemisphere where illness or injury damaged a person's ability to form words.

In Germany, Carl Wernicke borrowed from Broca's thinking and pinpointed the spot, also usually in the left hemisphere, that controlled coherent sentence construction. Berlin physiologist Eduard Hitzig and zoologist Gustav Fritsch discovered that by applying a mild electric shock to

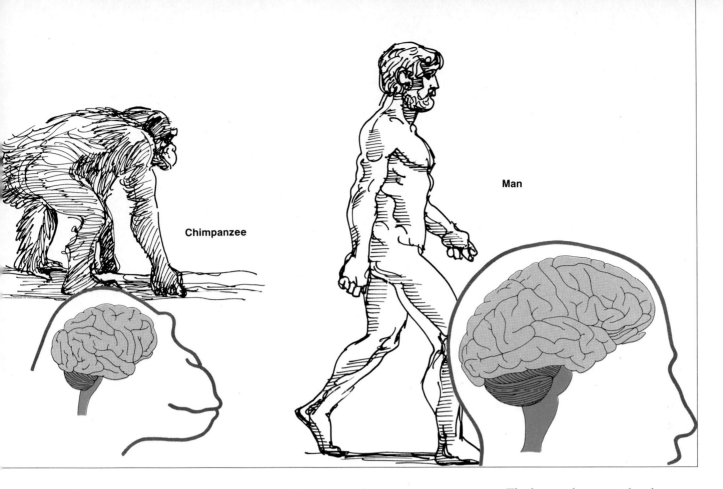

Chimpanzee

Man

the exposed cortex, "one gets combined muscle contractions of the opposite half of the body."

Scotsman David Ferrier, building on the research of Hitzig and Fritsch, mapped in detail the motor cortex and also located the parallel sensory strip. He found "no reason to suppose that one part of the brain is excitable and another not. The question is how the stimulation manifests itself." With electrodes and surgical knives he experimented on animals ranging from pigeons to monkeys, applying what he learned to observations in humans. He concluded that "mental operations, in the last analysis, must be merely the subjective side of sensory and motor substrata." Expressing the same idea in an evolutionary context, Ferrier's colleague, English neurologist John Hughlings Jackson, asserted that motor centers of the brain are the "climax of nervous evolution" and comprise the "organ of mind." He envisioned three evolutionary centers: the lowest, embracing brainstem components; the "middle centre;" and the highest, the motor and sensory areas of the cerebral cortex that he characterized as "the anatomical substrata of consciousness."

Jackson's definition of evolution as "a passage from the most automatic to the most voluntary" functional centers of the brain foreshadowed a

The human brain weighs about three pounds, dwarfing those of the other vertebrates portrayed above. The buff-colored cerebrum, source of human thought and creativity, occupies two-thirds of man's massive brain. Other than man, only mammals, represented by the cat and the chimpanzee, possess cerebrums of any size or complexity. In vertebrates lower than mammals, the cerebrum is tiny and takes up proportionately less of the brain's space.

Bearded Russian Ivan Pavlov would
ring a bell before feeding his dog.
Anticipating food, the dog's digestive system would respond every time
the bell rang. This physiological
response was a conditioned reflex.

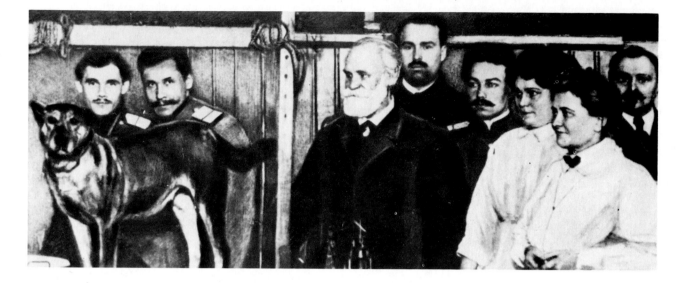

twentieth-century concept, the three-stage "tri-une" brain hypothesized by Paul MacLean of the National Institute of Mental Health. MacLean coined "reptilian" for the part Jackson labeled lowest, suggesting cold-blooded survival through basic drives. In MacLean's paleomammalian brain, corresponding to Jackson's middle center, wells emotion, the "affective feelings" typified by mammals nursing their young. MacLean's thinking neomammalian brain is equivalent to Jackson's highest centers. Strong neurological ties link the three brains together, says MacLean, enabling the more primitive structures to "temper reason with emotion." As Jackson put it three-quarters of a century earlier, "They are the unifying centres of the whole organism."

In nineteenth-century forums scholars argued whether the mind evolved with the brain or existed apart. Rallying around the latter view were followers of Immanuel Kant, Prussian professor of logic and metaphysics who declared, "No experience tells me that I am shut up in some place in my brain." Charles Darwin, controversial theorist of evolution, could not resist the argument; he took the pragmatic view. "Why," Darwin reasoned, "is thought being a secretion of the brain more wonderful than gravity a property of matter?" Was there a middle ground to this "world knot," as Schopenhauer termed the impasse between mind and matter? Nobel Prize-winning

physiologist C. S. Sherrington thought so, theorizing that "the brain and the psyche lie together, so to say, on a knife's edge" — or on the tip of a satirist's tongue:

"What is mind?"
"No matter."
"What is matter?"
"Never mind."

No laughing matter were the experiments that Ivan Pavlov conducted in Russia. He trained dogs to salivate by stimulating their nervous systems with bells and electricity. After watching one of Pavlov's hungry dogs endure hot probes to get meat, then salivate when the electrodes were applied and the meat withdrawn, Sherrington exclaimed: "At last I understand the psychology of the martyrs!"

Making the mind behave challenged Johns Hopkins psychologist John Watson in the early 1900s. Believing that action stimulated thought and not vice versa, he used Pavlov's conditioned-reflex mechanism as the basic building block of all learning, making it the cornerstone of a theory he called behaviorism. He held that thought was simply speech unuttered, that "there is no such thing as an inheritance of capacity, talent, temperament, mental constitution and characteristics." Given a dozen healthy babies and his own special environment, Watson guaranteed "to take

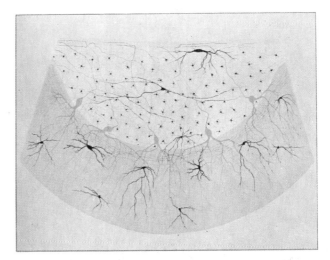

any one at random and train him to become any kind of specialist I might select — doctor, lawyer, beggarman and thief." George Bernard Shaw pursued this theme in the play *Pygmalion*, his professor Henry Higgins teaching cockney flower girl Eliza Doolittle the speech and manners of a well-bred English lady.

Sharing the stage with behaviorists were the interpreters of the mind. Foremost among them stood Sigmund Freud, the Viennese father of psychoanalysis. He sought the innermost thoughts of his patients to learn "how the mental apparatus is constructed and what forces interplay and counteract in it."

While Freud and his followers wrestled with the mind, others devised methods to penetrate the brain's substance. "In the intricate warp of the brain one can advance only step by step," wrote Spain's Santiago Ramón y Cajal. He and Camillo Golgi shared a Nobel Prize in 1906 for the most important milestone in neuroanatomy since the development of the microscope. Golgi devised a way to selectively stain nerve tissue. Ramón y Cajal later disproved Golgi's idea that cells formed an interlocking network.

Using Golgi's staining technique under the microscope, he proved that each nerve cell was a distinct body consisting of nucleus and branching tendrils. One, the axon, transmitted information; the others, dendrites, received. Other scientists would soon discover that nerve cells communicated through electrical and chemical pulses at infinitesimal junctions called synapses. Descartes would have recognized the system immediately: a nerve machine.

With today's technology, neuroscientists examine brain tissue for clues to such phenomena as nerve regeneration and sprouting of neural fibers. Does the brain explain the mind, wondered neurosurgeon Wilder Penfield, "by the simple performance of its neuronal mechanisms, or by supplying energy to the mind? Or both?" Brain surgeon Roger Sperry of the California Institute of Technology concluded that the brain's consciousness encompassed and transcended its physical workings: "In the human head there are forces within forces within forces, as in no other cubic half-foot of the universe that we know."

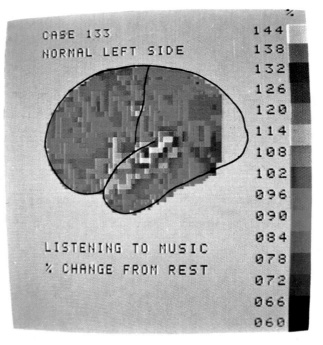

CASE 133
NORMAL LEFT SIDE

LISTENING TO MUSIC
% CHANGE FROM REST

%
144
138
132
126
120
114
108
102
096
090
084
078
072
066
060

Sounds of music register white, red and yellow on this brain scan. Radioactive isotopes injected into arteries enable blood flow to be measured, locating areas of increased activity in the cortex.

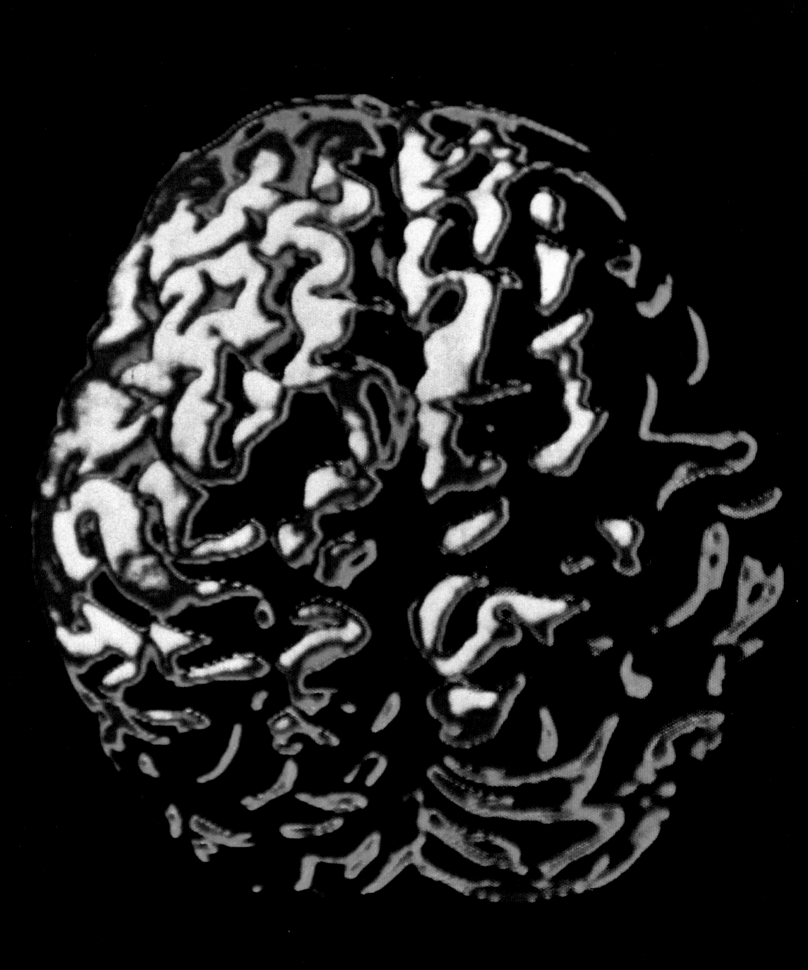

Chapter 2

Landscapes of the Brain

"The citadel of sense-perception," Roman scholar Pliny the Elder defined the brain. "Thoroughfare for all thoughts," echoed Keats. Bathed in photography's expressionist hues, its furrowed crust of tissue teems with billions of cells. Deep fissures demarcate cerebral lobes. A cranial canyon, the longitudinal sulcus, divides left and right hemispheres.

As long as the brain is a mystery," declared nineteenth-century anatomist Ramón y Cajal, "the universe . . . will also be a mystery." From civilization's first dawning, the contemplative brain of man has probed for answers within itself as well as in the heavens. The earliest description of a human brain, found on a scroll of papyrus copied about 1600 B.C., tells of an Egyptian physician who reached into a shattered skull, a warrior's perhaps, and felt the brain "throbbing and fluttering under thy fingers." Roughly the size and shape of an athlete's fist, the pinkish gray brain weighs about three pounds. Yet appearance gives no clue to its limits. Ultimate enigma, the brain perplexes all who presume to take its measure.

Through the centuries surveyors of the brain charted every cerebral hill and valley. They sprinkled Latin names across the brainscape — corpus callosum, arbor vitae, hippocampus. They painstakingly analyzed functions of minute parts, seeking clues to sources of sensibility and motivation. Several structural concepts emerged. One divided the brain into three sections — forebrain, midbrain, hindbrain. Another theory assigned it three stages of evolution — reptilian, paleomammalian, neomammalian. Observers also determined the skull housed not one brain but two — a matched pair.

Two brains are better than one, as are two lungs and two hands. But a single hemisphere of the brain will suffice. The realization that one side has the capacity to perform independently of the other has long intrigued scientists. Nearly twenty-five hundred years ago, Hippocrates, patriarch of physicians, noted that a wound to the left side of the head affected only the right side of the body, and vice versa. He wisely concluded that "the brain of man is double."

Though symmetrical, the hemispheres are not necessarily equal. In most persons, the left brain

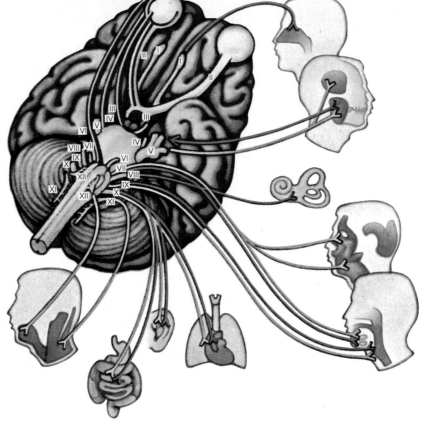

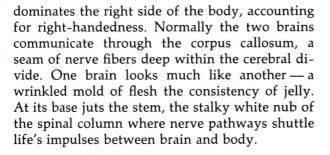

Twelve pairs of cranial nerves branch from the brainstem, sending sensory (purple) and motor (orange) fibers to head and body organs. Spot illustrations (clockwise from top) show nasal path of olfactory nerve; trigeminal nerve endings in chewing muscles and sensory facial areas; acoustic-nerve connections to the inner ear; facial-nerve motor fibers to face and scalp, sensory fibers from taste buds; wide-ranging vagus-nerve involvement in eardrum, lungs and stomach; and spinal-accessory nerve fibers that control head and shoulder movement; hypoglossal nerve leads to tongue.

dominates the right side of the body, accounting for right-handedness. Normally the two brains communicate through the corpus callosum, a seam of nerve fibers deep within the cerebral divide. One brain looks much like another — a wrinkled mold of flesh the consistency of jelly. At its base juts the stem, the stalky white nub of the spinal column where nerve pathways shuttle life's impulses between brain and body.

Survival and Sentience

The fibrous first inch of the brainstem contains the medulla oblongata. Its reflex centers, clusters of nerve cells called neurons, control heartbeat, blood pressure and breathing. From them flash signals to swallow, sneeze, laugh. Intolerant of injury or disease, the medulla has been called "the most vital part of the entire brain." It is the evolutionary core, the primitive site for survival in man or lizard.

More than a control center, the medulla also serves as the crossroads for nerve tracts binding body and brain. Sensory nerves from trunk and limbs switch lanes with motor nerves that originate in the brain's wrinkled thinking cap, the cerebral cortex. Distinctive medulla landmarks include the pyramidal decussation where nerve

fibers bunch in front, and the inferior olivary nuclear complex, gray masses of olive-shaped cells bulging from the sides.

Guarding the rear of the medulla is the reticular formation, a thimble-sized web of interlocking neuron circuits. Within this tangle ticks the brain's alarm apparatus, monitoring the sensory signals that pass through. The smell of smoke would instantly set off the reticular formation alarm, alerting the decision-making cortex to start its neuron motors. Without that silent warning, wrote the neurophysiologist John D. French, a person would be "reduced to a helpless, senseless, paralyzed blob of protoplasm."

From the medulla and adjacent areas radiate the twelve pairs of cranial nerves. They serve the sensory and motor needs of head, neck, chest and abdomen. Counting from front to back, top to bottom, the twelve are known by both name and Roman numeral: olfactory (I), optic (II), oculomotor (III), trochlear (IV), trigeminal (V), abducens (VI), facial (VII), acoustic (VIII), glossopharyngeal (IX), vagus (X), spinal accessory (XI) and hypoglossal (XII). To remember them in order, anatomy students key on the first letter of each name and recite: "On old Olympus's tiny tops a Finn and German viewed some hops."

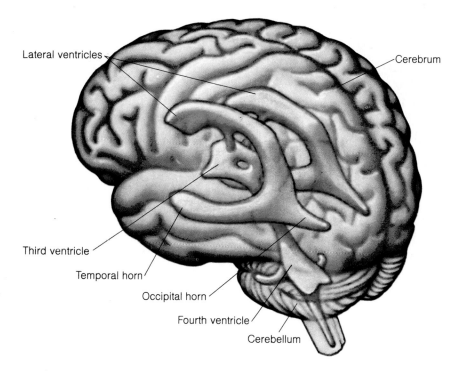

Lateral ventricles

Cerebrum

Third ventricle

Temporal horn

Occipital horn

Fourth ventricle

Cerebellum

Limpid pools of cerebrospinal fluid bathe the brain and cushion it against shock. Secreted from choroid tissue resembling tiny egg clusters, the plasmalike fluid fills four cranial cavities, the ventricles. From the low fourth ventricle, the fluid circulates through shallows around the brain and down the spinal cord.

Another view is from the bridge — the pons, as sixteenth-century anatomist Costanzo Varoli dubbed it. Arching over the medulla, this inch-wide span of white matter ribbed with fibers serves as a neuronal link between cerebral cortex and cerebellum, the fore- and hindbrains. From the bridge itself extends a third of the cranial nerves, including the largest, the trigeminal. As the name suggests, this nerve cable branches into three pairs, with sensory fibers fanning out to jaws, scalp and face. Trigeminal endings in the nose are sensitive to ammonia-based substances like smelling salts. A single whiff jangles the consciousness-restoring impulses of the pontine reticular formation, extending up from the medulla. In the same vicinity is the reticulated control center that regulates breathing rhythm.

Washing against Varoli's bridge is the fourth ventricle, modest reservoir — a scant spoonful — of the brain's precious cerebrospinal fluid. Springing from capillary membranes, the clear, plasmalike liquid trickles into mirrored lateral ventricles, seeps down into the third ventricle, and flows through the narrow cerebral aqueduct into the fourth ventricle. From this shining pool, angled like a diamond, the fluid circulates upward into spongy subarachnoid spaces of the

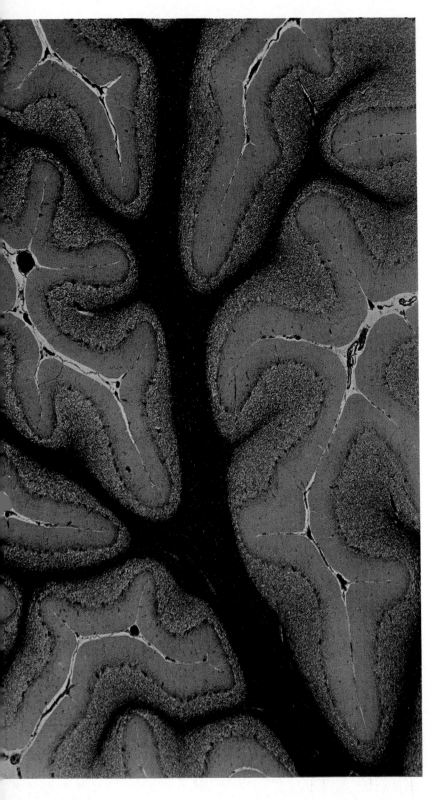

*Arbor vitae, medieval anatomists'
"tree of life," patterns a cross-
section of the cerebellum. This
"lesser brain" below the cerebrum
coordinates muscle movement and
helps control balance and posture.*

brain and downward into the spine. Drained of its nutrients and laden with metabolic wastes, the liquid is reabsorbed into the blood. Renewed about three times a day, the supply measures less than half a pint. But that is enough to fill the ventricular lakes and all their tributaries.

Harmony in Movement

Beyond the fourth ventricle rise the rumpled gray hills of the cerebellum. Wedged between stem and cerebral hemispheres, it forms a distinct body — a protoplasmic subcontinent accounting for almost an eighth of the brain's mass. Called the "lesser brain" for its cortex and core, the cerebellum governs a human's every movement. Apparently initiating nothing itself, the cerebellum monitors impulses from motor centers in the brain and from nerve endings in muscles. Modifying and coordinating commands to swing or sway, it grooves a golfer's tee shot, smoothes a dancer's footwork or, more typically, lets a hand glide glass to lips without sloshing the contents.

In evolutionary growth, it has been calculated that over the past million years the cerebellum has more than tripled in size. Theoretically, it is still growing. Muscular skills, it follows, should keep pace, and Olympic records suggest they do. There is evidence the cerebellum may also play a role in a person's emotional development, modulating sensations of pleasure and anger.

Opened like a book, the cerebellum reveals facing pages of a striking foliate pattern. *Arbor vitae,* medieval anatomists labeled it — the tree of life. They pondered its meaning, seeking in its branches the source of the soul.

The branching results from deep folds in the cerebellar cortex, so wrinkled that 85 percent of its surface remains hidden. This thick skin of gray matter comprises three layers of cells and fibers, the middle layer consisting of Purkinje cells, named after the Czech physiologist who first described them in 1837. Treelike themselves with myriad forking tendrils called dendrites, Purkinje cells rank among the most complex of all neurons. One cell's dendrites may receive nerve information from a hundred thousand fibers through wispy contact points called synapses. No other kind of cell in the entire nervous system makes as many synaptic connections. These trigger a response in the Purkinje dispatcher — an inhibitor, by nature — which flashes instructions to the white matter of the arbor vitae, then to other points in the brain and body.

Close the cerebellum and the botanical image vanishes. The paired lobes assume the silhouette of a moth. Between the "wings" curls a grublike section called the vermis, which helps to maintain balance, tone muscles, control posture.

From either side of the vermis protrude three cerebellar feet, the peduncles. Through them shuttle nerve impulses from incoming and outgoing fibers. The incoming afferents outnumber the departing efferents three to one. Afferents enter the cerebellum mainly through two pairs of peduncles, which connect respectively to medulla and pons. Most of the efferent fibers, stemming from cell nuclei deep inside the cerebellum, weave through the twin superior peduncles. Over them speed messages — like "easy does it" — as peduncular paths cross at the base of the midbrain, tunnel into pink-tinted gray matter called the red nucleus, wend upward into the thalamus and connect there to the cortex.

Beyond Midbrain's End

It is a short trip through the midbrain — less than an inch. From its back side jut four little hills, the colliculi, which serve as relay stations for sound and sight impulses. Straddling the midbrain front are peduncles from above, cerebral peninsulas veined with descending fibers destined for faraway places in the trunk and limbs.

Down the peduncle core courses a thick layer of dark cellular matter stained with the pigment melanin. This is the substantia nigra, mother lode of the biochemical agent dopamine, which guards against muscle rigidity and tremor.

Wondrous alchemy is produced in the remote enclaves beyond midbrain's end. In this region surrounding the third ventricle lies the hypothalamus, synthesizer of hormones to control growth, raise and lower temperature, regulate the body's water balance and activate sexual behavior. These hormones funnel into the pituitary gland, an island nerve center in itself, where they are stored or released into the bloodstream.

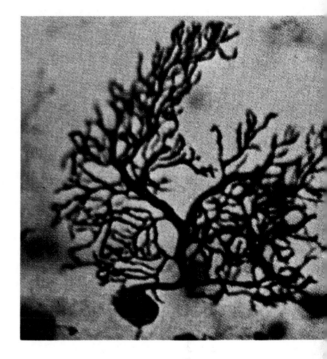

Fernlike Purkinje cells lace the folded cortex of the cerebellum. Branching dendrites of a single cell make thousands of contacts with other fibers, forming one of the most complex information-gathering systems in the brain. The cell body dispatches messages through a lone, trailing axon.

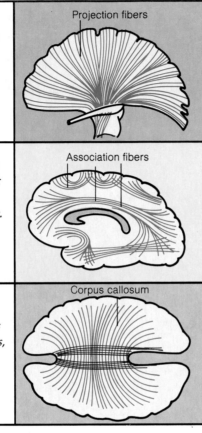

Projection fibers
Forming the corona radiata, *these fibers fan out from the brainstem. They relay impulses to and from the cortex.*

Projection fibers

Association fibers
Looping strands link different sections of the same hemisphere. This web subtly modulates the cerebral cortex.

Association fibers

Corpus callosum
This thicket of fibers joins the hemispheres, permitting the two sides of the brain to communicate with each other.

Corpus callosum

Electrical as well as chemical activity powers hypothalamic generators, cell masses specializing in involuntary behavior control. These centers crackle with energy as they light up circuits signaling the body to eat, drink, get angry, keep cool, make love. All that power and more fits into a quarter-ounce lump of gray matter.

To the rear, from the roof of the third ventricle, projects the pea-sized pineal gland. Once thought to be the vestige of a primitive third eye — as in a frog — the pineal gland may in fact be a light-activated biological clock that regulates sex-gland activity.

The two thalami, side-by-side domes at the top of the brainstem, help to regulate consciousness. Gray masses packed in the domes gather information from nearly every area of the body, relaying sensory impulses to the cerebrum above.

Paired limbic lobes, joined at the top by a fibrous web called the fornix, ring the hubs of the thalamus. The limbic system is the "emotional brain." Sensory pathways of smell share limbic rights of way with memory lanes and the hairpin turns of raw emotion. Sensations of ecstasy and agony travel these routes, entering and exiting the cerebrum, cerebellum and other way stations. Neurophysiologist Paul MacLean cites "its central role in generating affective feelings, including those important for a sense of reality . . . and a conviction of what is true and important."

Arranged symmetrically in the brain, the two lateral ventricles form a pattern that, looking up from the brainstem, suggests a prehistoric bird in flight. Above spreads the vaulted cerebrum, the two-thirds of the brain where human thought and creativity originate. "Wider than the sky" it seemed to poet Emily Dickinson, who disdained its coarse measure. Still wider than man's understanding, it reveals its mystery in grudging bits.

The Dual Brain

The wide spaces of the cerebrum house white matter, masses of fibers sheathed in fatty fabric. These hundreds of millions of microscopic threads form an array of connections between the cortex's nerve centers and distant parts of the brain. Projection fibers, one of three cerebral classifications, squeeze into a compact band called the internal capsule, located near the top of the brainstem. The fibers, both incoming and outgoing, flare to all parts of the cerebral cortex, creating a scalloped pattern anatomists dubbed corona radiata. Association fibers, the most numerous, remain within hemispheric limits, providing each side of the brain with built-in self-sufficiency. One of the association skeins, the cingulum, loops over the corpus callosum.

The corpus callosum, that four-inch-long body of densely packed commissural fibers, is the third category, knitting together the cerebral hemispheres. Extending beyond the brain's midline, its strands bridge the lateral ventricles and, intermingling with association and projection fibers, radiate to most areas of the cortex.

The corpus callosum connection has long intrigued scientists. Its massive size and central location led them to believe it essential to the brain's proper functioning. The great cerebral

Roger Sperry

Probing the Two Minds of Man

In the late 1930s, neurosurgeons hoping to control severe epileptic seizures in some of their patients first took the radical step of severing the corpus callosum — the largest neural bridge between the hemispheres of the brain. In some patients, the seizures stopped completely after surgery. More remarkably, the patients showed virtually no other obvious changes in personality, capacities or behavior.

Medical science had long thought the corpus callosum to be one of the major pathways of the brain. But if severing this massive neural connection had no influence on temperament or behavior, why did it exist at all?

In the early 1960s, psychobiologist Roger Sperry and his colleagues at the California Institute of Technology began trying to solve this riddle by testing "split-brain" patients. In eventually solving it they uncovered an even greater mystery — the mystery of man's two minds.

Sperry and his colleagues designed special tests to probe the functions of the divided brain. A split-brain patient would be seated in front of a screen on which images could be flashed to either side of his brain. Another screen hid the

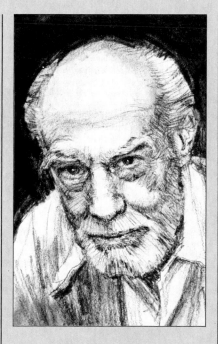

patient's hands from his view. As in virtually all right-handed people, the dominant left hemisphere of the patient's brain controlled both the right side of his body and his speech centers. If the researchers placed a familiar object, say, a spoon, in the patient's right hand, he could easily name it. But if they put the spoon in his left hand, he could only guess at what he held.

In another test, the researchers flashed different figures to the two sides of the subject's brain — a dollar sign to the left side, for example, and a question mark to the right. They then asked the patient to

use his left hand to draw what he had just seen. He drew a question mark. Asked what he had just drawn, he said without hesitation, "a dollar sign."

One side of a subject's brain, in some tests, would scold the other with a frown or a scowl for an incorrect answer. One patient complained of a "sinister left hand" that untied his robe as his right hand tried to tie it or pulled off his trousers as his right hand struggled to pull them on.

In Sperry's words, each hemisphere of the divided brain "seems to have its own separate and private sensations; its own perceptions; its own impulses to act, with related volitional, cognitive and learning experiences."

Sperry and his colleagues proved that an intricate division of labor exists in the brain, and in doing so they solved the riddle of the corpus callosum. It exists largely to unify attention and awareness and allow the two hemispheres to share learning and memory. But this solution presents all who would know the brain with a more profound mystery. If the corpus callosum links a divided brain, does it also link a divided mind? And if the mind is divided, how is it divided — for or against itself, or both?

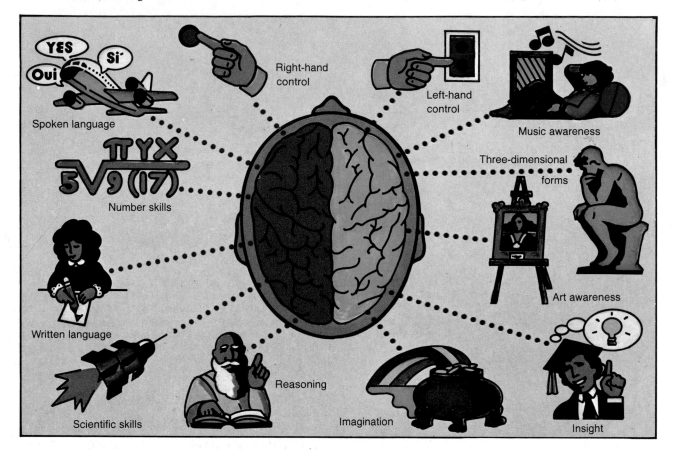

commissure, as they termed it, clearly united the two halves of the mental self. "All its diversity is merged into oneness," asserted physiologist Sir Charles Sherrington. But evidence gleaned over the past century and a half suggests that mental unity may be more illusory than real.

The notion that a person could function with a single cerebral hemisphere first dawned in the mid-nineteenth century. A. L. Wigan, a British physician, performed autopsies on men who had apparently led normal lives with only half a brain. Wigan reasoned that if one hemisphere were "capable of all the emotions, sentiments and faculties which we call in the aggregate, mind — then it necessarily follows that Man must have two minds with two brains."

A century later, surgeons discovered that cutting the corpus callosum inhibited the severity of epileptic seizures. Surprisingly, the surgery caused no noticeable impairment of normal be-

havior. One patient, his sense of humor still intact, wryly complained of a "splitting headache."

In the 1950s, split-brain research conducted by the California Institute of Technology's Roger Sperry and colleagues proved that the corpus callosum united the special powers of both hemispheres. Their sight and touch tests demonstrated that man was unquestionably of two minds, one specializing in analytical and verbal skills, the other adept in space and pattern perception. The left hemisphere dealt in the abstract symbols of language and numbers. It was logical, linear, fragmentary and sequential in processing information. The left hemisphere sorted out parts. The right hemisphere grasped things as a whole. It generated mental images of sight, sound, touch, taste and smell, comparing relationships. It was holistic and simultaneous in its thinking.

Sperry's studies established that the brain divided can function as ably as the brain intact.

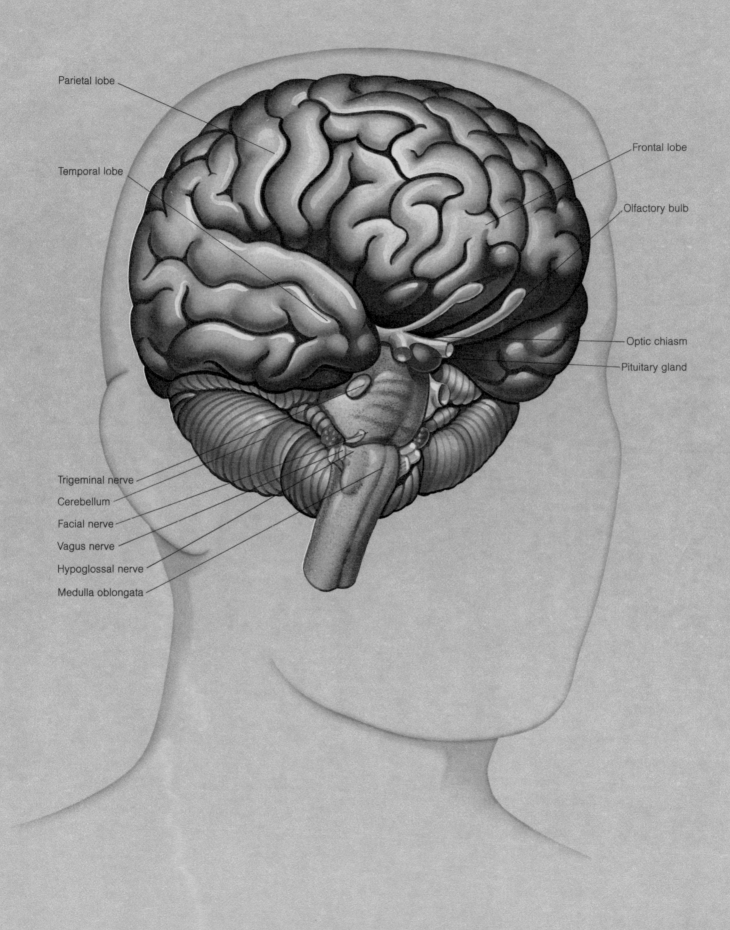

Parietal lobe

Temporal lobe

Frontal lobe

Olfactory bulb

Optic chiasm

Pituitary gland

Trigeminal nerve

Cerebellum

Facial nerve

Vagus nerve

Hypoglossal nerve

Medulla oblongata

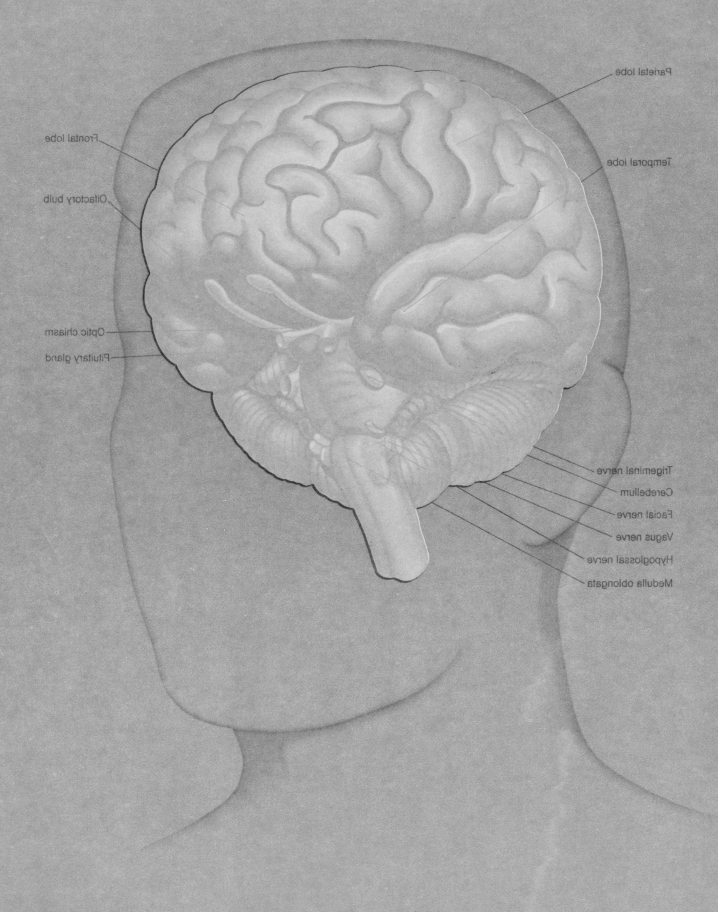

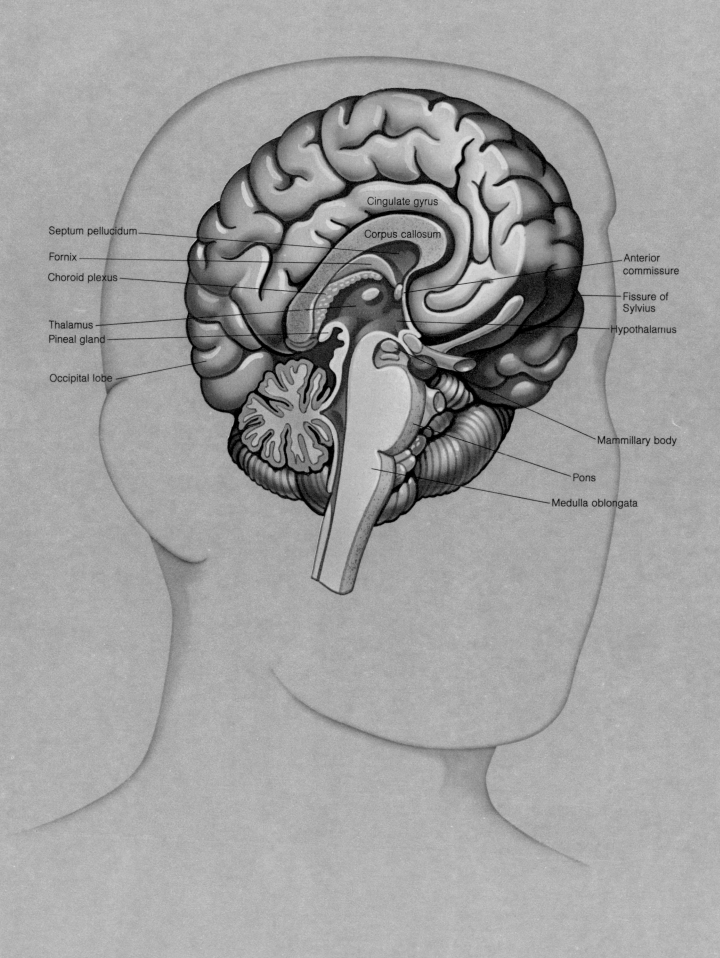

Septum pellucidum

Fornix

Choroid plexus

Thalamus

Pineal gland

Occipital lobe

Cingulate gyrus

Corpus callosum

Anterior commissure

Fissure of Sylvius

Hypothalamus

Mammillary body

Pons

Medulla oblongata

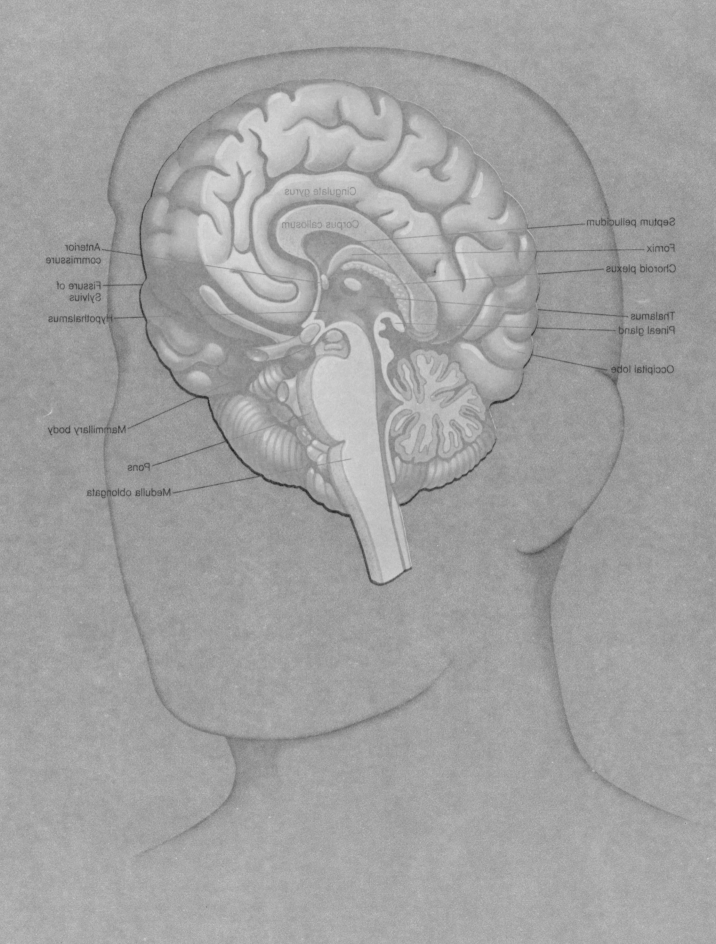

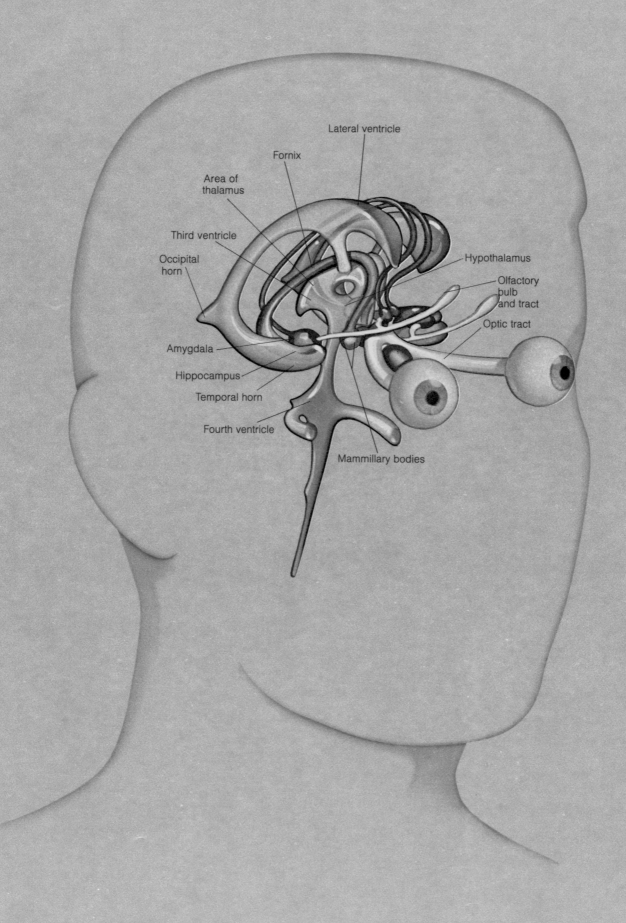

Lateral ventricle

Fornix

Area of
thalamus

Third ventricle

Occipital
horn

Hypothalamus

Olfactory
bulb
and tract

Optic tract

Amygdala

Hippocampus

Temporal horn

Fourth ventricle

Mammillary bodies

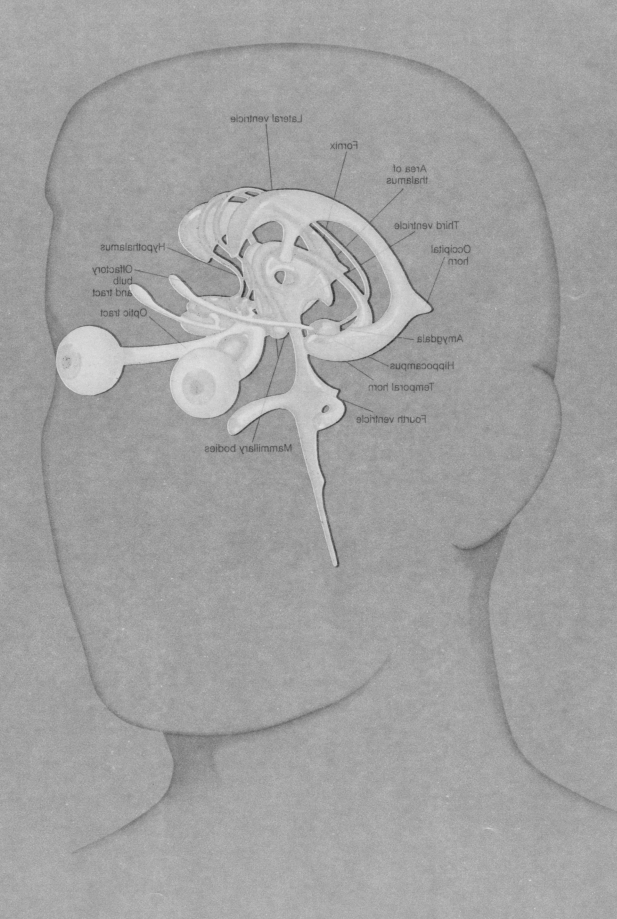

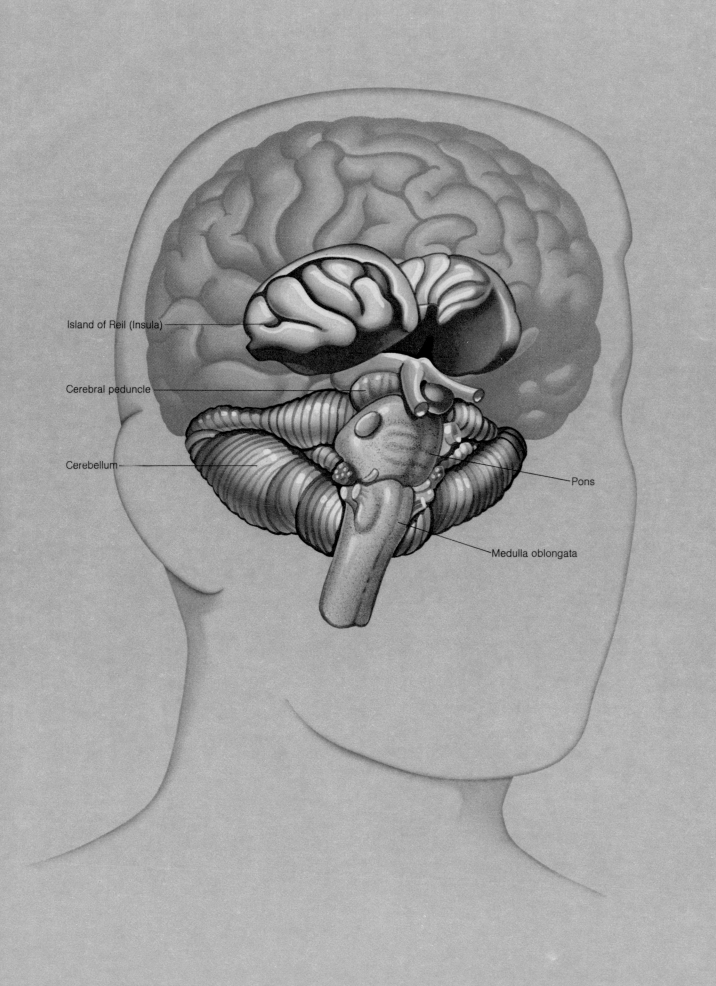

Island of Reil (Insula)

Cerebral peduncle

Cerebellum

Pons

Medulla oblongata

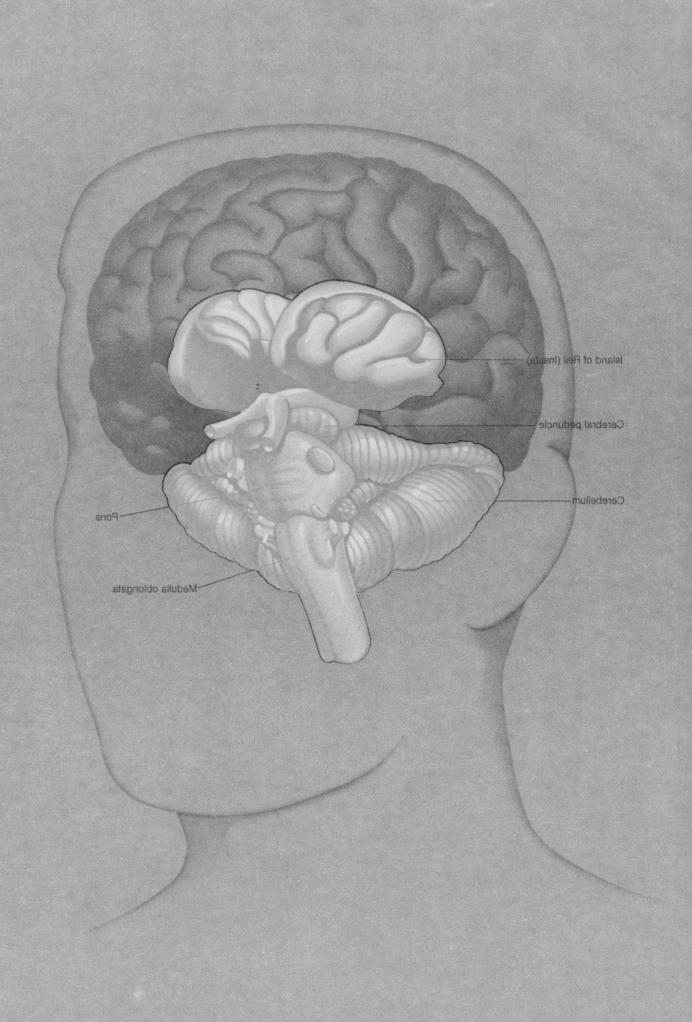

Medulla oblongata

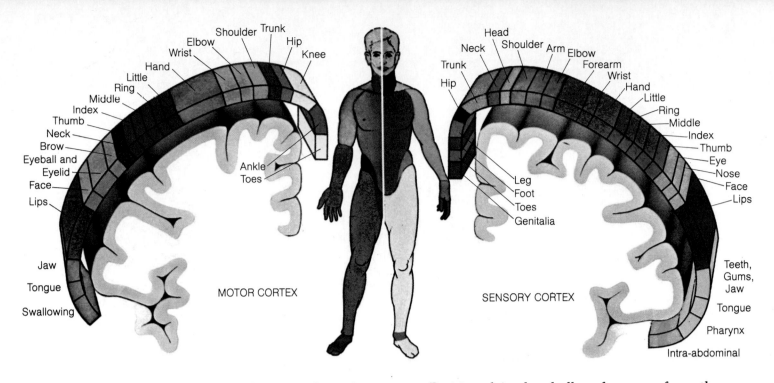

MOTOR CORTEX

SENSORY CORTEX

Bisected-brain patients have performed two tasks while normal persons completed one. Splitting the brain seems to result in two spheres of consciousness. Echoing Wigan, Sperry saw in a bisected brain "two separate 'selves' — essentially a divided organism, each with its own memories and its own will — competing for control."

Man's Temporal Heavens

Most of what they vie to control originates in the gray matter of the cerebral cortex. Less than a quarter-inch thick, it forms a fissured mold snug against the skull. The cortex measures about two-and-a-half square feet, roughly twice the expanse of this book opened, and weighs twenty ounces or so. This "bark" of flesh is composed of six layers of cells meshed in some ten thousand miles of connecting fibers per cubic inch. About ten billion pyramidal, spindle and stellate cells spangle the cortex like twinkling galaxies.

Mapping this temporal heaven, man blocked out four areas on each side of the brain's longitudinal sulcus. This front-to-rear cleft divides the two hemispheres above the corpus callosum. Forward of the central fissure, angling downward from the top of the cortex toward the ear, curves the frontal lobe. Massed within the gyri, or folds, are batteries of motor neurons ready to fire. They control every voluntary movement from a handshake to the wink of an eye. Sensory cells that respond to touch, heat, cold, pain and body position cluster in parallel ribbons of nerve tissue behind the central fissure. This area, the parietal lobe, caps the back of the cerebral cortex.

Positioned in the skull as far away from the eyes as possible, the visual cortex occupies an area in the occipital lobe, at the back of each hemisphere. From the retinas, light-triggered impulses race over the million fibers of the optic nerve, half of them crossing at the chiasma junction in front of the brainstem. They fan out through paired cell clusters called lateral geniculate bodies and, traveling at speeds of up to 400 feet per second, slam into the occipital cell bank, stimulating the miracle of seeing. Hearing is processed in the temporal lobe, delineated from the frontal by the lateral fissure at sideburn level.

While sound and light stimulate sensory and motor areas, stimulation of the association cortex is much more complex. Here, spanning regions of both the frontal and temporal lobes, dwell the mysteries of thought, memory and language.

Two language-control areas were charted more than a century ago by neurologists Pierre Paul Broca and Carl Wernicke. Broca's area wedges between the lateral fissure and the lower portion of the motor cortex, which controls muscles of the face and throat. Below the lateral fissure and next to the sensory cortex is Wernicke's area. Together, they direct the smooth transfer of thought and expression into speech.

Long ago, physicians realized that locating the sources of speech and language disorder presented two different challenges. They found that tissue damage in the Broca and Wernicke areas of the left hemisphere did not necessarily cause permanent impairment of normal speech. Linguistic functions may be assumed by other areas, in-

Spanning the brain like earphones, adjacent bands of cortex trigger motion and register sensations. Diagram, opposite, maps sensory and motor cortexes, associating areas with various parts of the body.

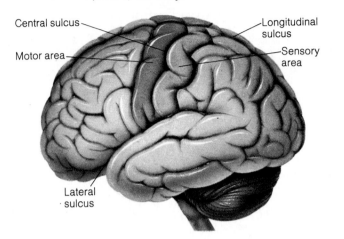

Central sulcus

Longitudinal sulcus

Motor area

Sensory area

Lateral sulcus

Wired for action, the motor cortex sends impulses along nerve fiber tracts. Most cross in the medulla before entering the spinal cord, fibers from the left activating muscles on the right and vice versa.

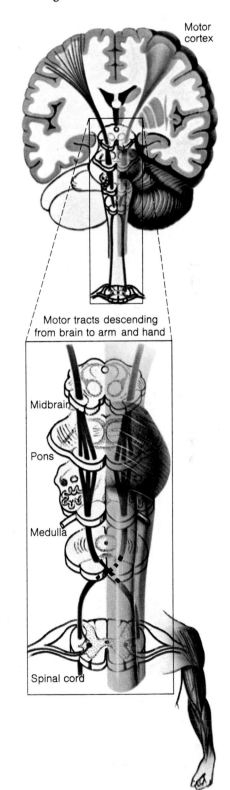

Motor cortex

Motor tracts descending from brain to arm and hand

Midbrain

Pons

Medulla

Spinal cord

cluding those in the right hemisphere, dormant until compelling need awakens lazy neurons.

Sperry saw in one hemisphere's dominance of speaking and writing skills "a belated tendency in evolution to try to circumvent some of the duplication difficulties." In instances where both hemispheres have dominant speech capabilities, stammering and other language difficulties seem to result.

Is the brain still evolving — and, if so, where? MacLean jested that the vaguely charted prefrontal cortex, realm of planning and foresight, might be a proper area for future evolution. And where in the brain resides the true self, neurosurgeon Joseph Bogen's "inner conviction of Oneness?" Where are the keys to the allegorical black box of the brain that holds the answers to the unknowns of evolution and creation? Could they be the same? We lack, says Sperry, "even a reasonable hypothesis" to comprehend the mental activities that cause a "simple volitional twitch of one's little finger."

Imagination's urging and scientists' skills permit the fearless exploring of cerebral landscapes. But because each explorer is tempted to seek within for intuitive direction, there can be no objectivity, no detached rationale. The poet Charles Churchill, having discovered this, cautioned the painter William Hogarth not to think too much about thinking.

> With curious art the brain,
> too finely wrought,
> Preys on herself, and is
> destroyed by thought.

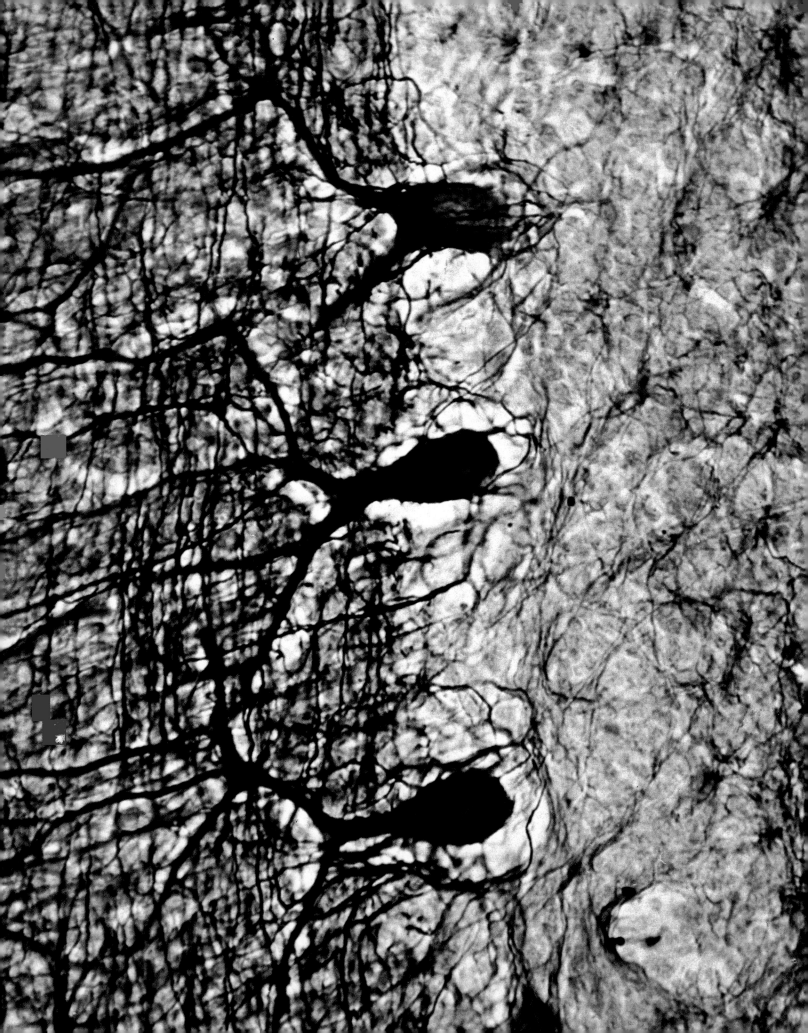

Chapter 3

The Electrochemical Brain

In Michelangelo's painting *The Creation of Adam*, the hands of God and Adam reach out to each other but do not touch as God gives Adam the divine spark, creating the soul of man. Within man's brain a similar event occurs. Billions upon billions of nerve cells in the human brain make perhaps as many as a quadrillion connections. As each nerve finger reaches toward another an earthly spark passes: an electrical and chemical impulse that enables us to think, feel, learn, remember, move and sense the world around us. Flashing in intricate patterns from one neuron to the next, this electrochemical spark somehow builds awareness, giving man the power to contemplate his own existence. It is indeed a spark of life.

Every nerve cell, or neuron, is a tiny information-processing system with thousands of connections through which it receives and sends signals. No two of these cells are exactly alike, but most share similar features: a cell body, dendrites and an axon. Inside the cell body are the nucleus and the biochemical machinery for maintaining the life of the cell. The dendrites, short fibers that extend from the cell body, branch out in the form of a bushy tree. Dendrites function as receivers, picking up impulses from neighboring nerve cells. The axon, one long fiber, extends from the cell body. At the end of the axon are tiny branches, each tipped with a small swelling, or terminal button. The axon serves as a transmitter, sending signals to other neurons.

Surrounding neurons are special cells known as glia. Outnumbering the neurons ten to one, the glial cells serve as packing material, gluing the brain together. They act as a buffer between the brain's blood vessels and the neurons, providing the nerve cells with nourishment and consuming waste products. They also insulate, separating each nerve cell from all others. Myelin, the special coating that protects long nerve fibers, comes

The warp and woof of the brain, slender nerve cells called neurons — here magnified 500 times — form a living fabric. Roughly 10 billion of them form the millimeters-thin cerebral cortex that gathers messages and sends commands signaling the body to respond.

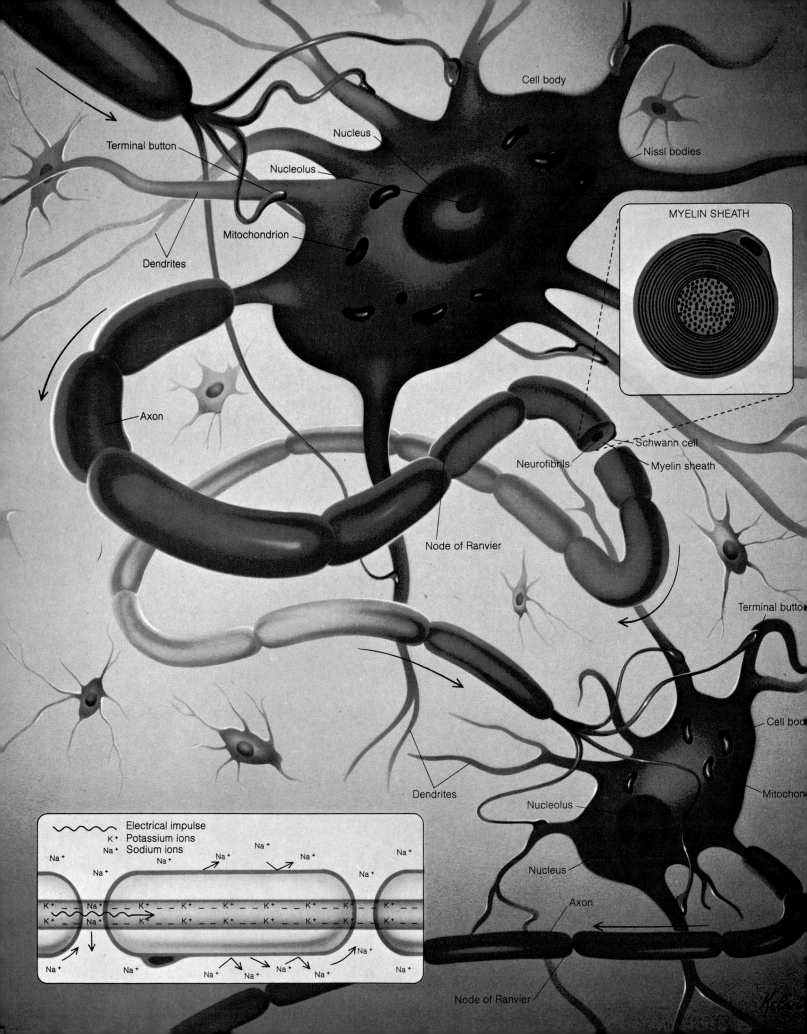

Cell body

Nucleus

Terminal button

Nucleolus

Nissl bodies

Mitochondrion

Dendrites

MYELIN SHEATH

Axon

Schwann cell

Neurofibrils

Myelin sheath

Node of Ranvier

Terminal button

Dendrites

Cell body

Mitochon

Nucleolus

Nucleus

Axon

Node of Ranvier

Electrical impulse
K + Potassium ions
Na + Sodium ions

Na +   Na +   Na +   Na +   Na +   Na +

Na +   Na +   Na +   Na +   Na +

K + — Na + — K + — K + — K + — K + — K + — K + — K +
K + — Na + — K + — K + — K + — K + — K + — K +

Na +   Na +   Na +   Na +   Na +   Na +   Na +

Billions of nerve cells similar to those below, direct the flow of information in the brain. Impulses entering the dendrites pass through the cell body and out along the axon. At axon's end, an impulse "fires"

neurotransmitters that flow out from the terminal button and across the synapse to a neighboring dendrite. Axons bundled into nerves, below right, thread through the spinal cord, connecting brain and body.

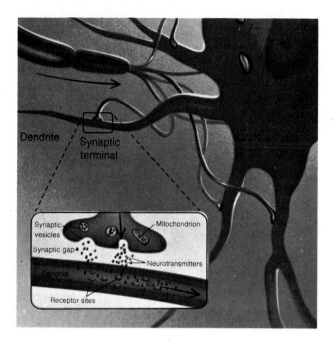

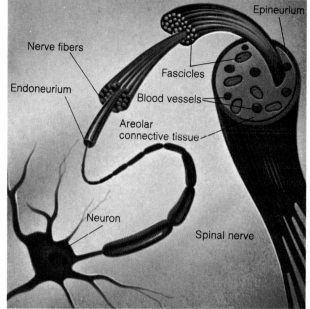

from glia. Since glial cells are sensitive to electricity, some scientists think they may serve as amplifiers, magnifying the faint electrical charges of nerve impulses. The only parts of neurons not covered by glial cells are the synapses, the junctions across which impulses travel from one nerve cell to another. The transmission of a nerve impulse is an electrochemical process. At the synapse the electrical impulses that travel through the cell convert into chemical signals, then back to electrical impulses.

In its resting state, the inside of a neuron has a slightly negative electrical charge compared to the outside. This is due to potassium ions, the electrically charged form of potassium atoms. The fluid outside the cell is high in positively charged sodium ions. When a neuron's dendrites pick up an impulse from a neighboring cell, a wave of electrical activity sweeps through the cell. If the impulse is strong enough, it will trigger a change in the axon's thin membrane, causing the cell to "fire." Special channels in the membrane open and sodium ions flow through, changing the internal charge of the membrane from negative to positive. Immediately other channels open, allowing potassium ions to flow out and restoring the negative internal voltage of

the membrane. This electrical relay race whips along the axon, turning the membrane positive, then negative again. So rapid is this transmission mechanism that in one one-thousandth of a second the axon is ready to carry another impulse.

At the end of the axon, the impulse strikes the terminal buttons, which contain tiny round sacs, or synaptic vesicles. The sacs burst open, spilling chemical messengers called neurotransmitters into the narrow synapse separating the terminal button from the next cell's dendrites. The neurotransmitters flow across the gap and lock onto receptor sites on the receiving cell's dendrites, sparking a second electrical current. Once it has passed on its signal, the neurotransmitter is destroyed by enzymes or recaptured and stored by the synaptic vesicles.

Not every cell contacted by neurotransmitters fires. A typical neuron may have one thousand to ten thousand synapses, receiving information from as many as a thousand other neurons. To avoid a tangled confusion of impulses, some synapses are inhibitory, tending to prevent the firing of the receiving cell. Synapses that promote a cell's firing are excitatory. A constant interplay between excitatory and inhibitory synapses determines whether a single neuron will fire.

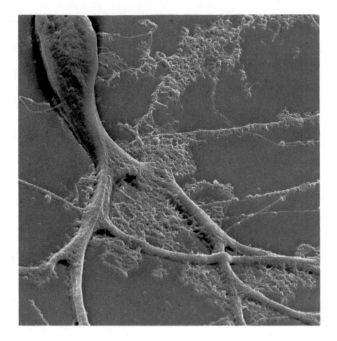

The fine mesh of nerve cell axons, dendrites and synaptic buttons link together in the brain. One cell (here at 20,000 times its size) can connect with 10,000 synapses, wiring it to perhaps a thousand other neurons.

All nerve cells use this process to transmit impulses. Axons of many nerve cells combine into cables to form nerve fibers. The direction of the impulse determines the function of a neuron. Sensory, or afferent, nerves carry messages from the body and the environment to the spinal cord and brain, which make up the central nervous system. Sensory neurons receive their information from receptors, special cells in sense organs, muscles, skin and joints. Interneurons found only in the brain and spinal cord pick up the afferent nerve impulses and relay them to motor nerves. Many serve an inhibitory function, helping to slow the flow of impulses flooding the brain. Motor, or efferent, neurons send the brain's responses back to muscles and glands.

This process can take place at incredible speeds. In some nerves, impulses travel more than 200 miles per hour. High-speed transmission occurs in neurons with wide axons and in those covered with a myelin sheath. This fatty coating insulates the neuron, leaving only small nodes, pinched points along the axon, exposed. The nerve impulses leap from node to node, enabling the brain to respond quickly to messages from the senses and the body.

Miraculous Migration

Understanding the way the brain works is as much a problem of form as of function. The story of the brain's structure begins at the start of life itself. Three weeks after conception, a single sheet of cells — no bigger than the tip of a paper match head — appears on the upper back of the human embryo. From this neural plate of a hundred thousand cells, the human brain folds itself into being. The plate curves into a groove, then closes into a tube. Furiously it grows, bulging here, elongating there, sprouting everywhere, at an average rate of 250,000 cells a minute.

As it grows, the neural tube divides. The upper part of the tube widens to form the ventricles, the cavities of the brain; and three major swellings appear, ultimately forming the forebrain, the midbrain and the hindbrain. The lower part of the tube develops into the spinal cord.

The walls of the neural tube thicken rapidly. The feverishly multiplying cells manufacture

Santiago Ramón y Cajal
Otto Loewi

Charting a Forest of Nerves

"The anatomy of the intimate structures of the brain is and remains apparently a book sealed with seven seals and written moreover in hieroglyphics," lamented a Viennese anatomist in 1846. More than forty years passed before Santiago Ramón y Cajal, a Spanish histologist, broke one of the seven seals. Searching for a method to reveal where one cell begins and another ends, he compared nerve tissue to a "forest so dense that . . . there are no spaces in it, so that the trunks, branches, and leaves touch everywhere."

His contemporaries were split between two theories of brain physiology: the reticular theory, which portrayed the brain as a continuous network of nerve fibers, with larger branches forming the spinal column — and the neuron doctrine, which held that the nervous system was composed of single nerve cells.

The "new truth," Ramón y Cajal reported, "laboriously sought and so elusive during two years of vain efforts, rose up suddenly in my mind like a revelation." Applying a new staining technique to the nerve cells of mammal embryos, he clearly saw under the microscope for the first time that each nerve cell was, in fact, an individual entity.

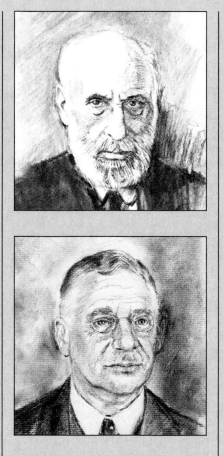

But the answer to one question raised another. If nerve cells were completely separate, how did they communicate? Scientists knew that nerves carried impulses in waves of electricity. They had assumed that nerve cells must pass the impulse from cell to cell through an electrical charge.

Yet, Austrian physiologist Otto Loewi proved that the process was not electrical, but chemical. One night in 1920, Loewi awoke from a dream and scribbled some notes on a piece of paper. But when he looked at the notes later that morning, they were indecipherable. The next night, his dream returned. Rather than risk losing the idea, he leapt out of bed and went straight to the laboratory.

Loewi filled one frog's heart with a saline solution and stimulated the nerve that slows the heartbeat. He then transferred the solution into another frog's heart in which that nerve had been severed. Magically, the heart's beating slowed. Here, he felt, was proof that the nerve secreted some chemical contained in the solution that controlled the frequency of heartbeat. That substance was later identified as the neurotransmitter acetylcholine.

Loewi made another observation likely shared by Ramón y Cajal, but one contrary to most notions of scientific research: "We should sometimes trust a sudden intuition without too much skepticism. If carefully considered in the daytime, I would undoubtedly have rejected the kind of experiment I performed. . . . It was good fortune that at the moment of the hunch I did not think but acted immediately."

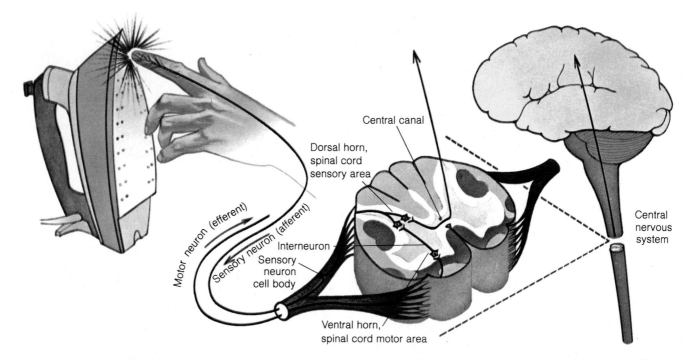

Central canal

Dorsal horn,
spinal cord
sensory area

Motor neuron (efferent)

Sensory neuron (afferent)

Interneuron

Sensory
neuron
cell body

Ventral horn,
spinal cord motor area

Central
nervous
system

A hot iron trips the body's reflex arc. The impulse moves straight from hand to spinal neurons and back to muscle, bypassing the brain to speed response. By the time the brain registers pain the hand has already recoiled.

life-encoding DNA in their nuclei. Flowing like amoebas, they migrate toward the center of the tube, thrusting out fat liquid tentacles and then drawing their nuclei after them. Along the inner surface of the tube they divide. Soon, the cells destined to become neurons exhaust their ability to make DNA, and dividing stops. The migrating cells obey such a precise biological timetable that neuroembryologists can predict a neuron's final destination in the brain by determining when it shuts down production of DNA. Glial cells retain the ability to divide throughout life.

But how does each neuron know where to go and what to do when it gets there? Experiments by Pasko Rakic of Yale University School of Medicine suggest that migrating neurons are guided to their destinations by a genetically imprinted roadmap. Specialized glial cells on the inner surface of the ventricles extend long tendrils to the neural tube wall where the neurons are multiplying. Rakic's studies have shown that the migrating neuron wraps itself around the glial tentacle and uses it as a road to travel inward.

Upon reaching their destinations, similar neurons link up to form specific brain regions and structures. The cells actually seem to recognize each other. Each neuron bears on its surface large identifying molecules, like so many I.D. badges, enabling each cell to find its proper companions. These marking molecules may also determine the order in which neurons link up, as well as the number and types of synaptic connections they make. Scientists suggest that most of the connections form during the brain's early development.

Models for Circuitry

In mapping the wiring of the brain, scientists found that some sensory messages require such a rapid response that they never even reach the brain. Touching a hot iron can trigger a protective circuit known as a reflex arc. When the hand touches the iron, receptor cells in the skin pick up the message and transmit it to sensory neurons which relay it directly to a motor neuron in the spinal cord. The motor nerve speeds a message back to the muscles of the arm and hand, which yank the fingers away.

The awareness of pain takes slightly longer; the finger has already left the iron by the time the burn is felt. As with the reflex arc, receptor cells send impulses to sensory nerves, which relay the impulses through the spinal cord to the brain. The sensation of the hot iron is one of many impulses going to the brain. Messages are constantly arriving from all parts of the body. The brain weighs the importance of all incoming impulses, acting first on the most urgent. The strong sensation of a burned finger will override lesser sensations as the brain calls into action a web of motor neurons which, in turn, trigger the muscular responses of a frown and a cry of pain.

Scientists are still trying to unravel the intricate interactions that enable man to reason and create. Modern theories attempt to explain the brain's more complex circuitry by creating a model for the movement and processing of nerve impulses. Nobel Prize-winning immunologist Gerald Edelman finds similarities between the brain and the immune system. Both are powerful recognition systems, thinks Edelman, able to "name or tag an object uniquely." Both are able to store that information for future reference. Yet neither has encountered the information before. "The central problem for the organism," he says, "is to classify things it could not have known."

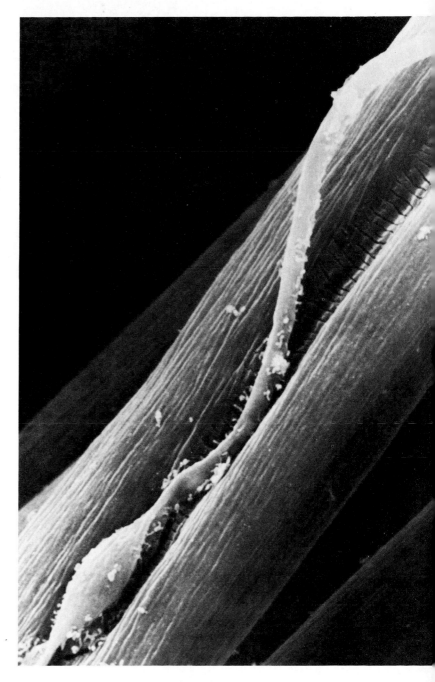

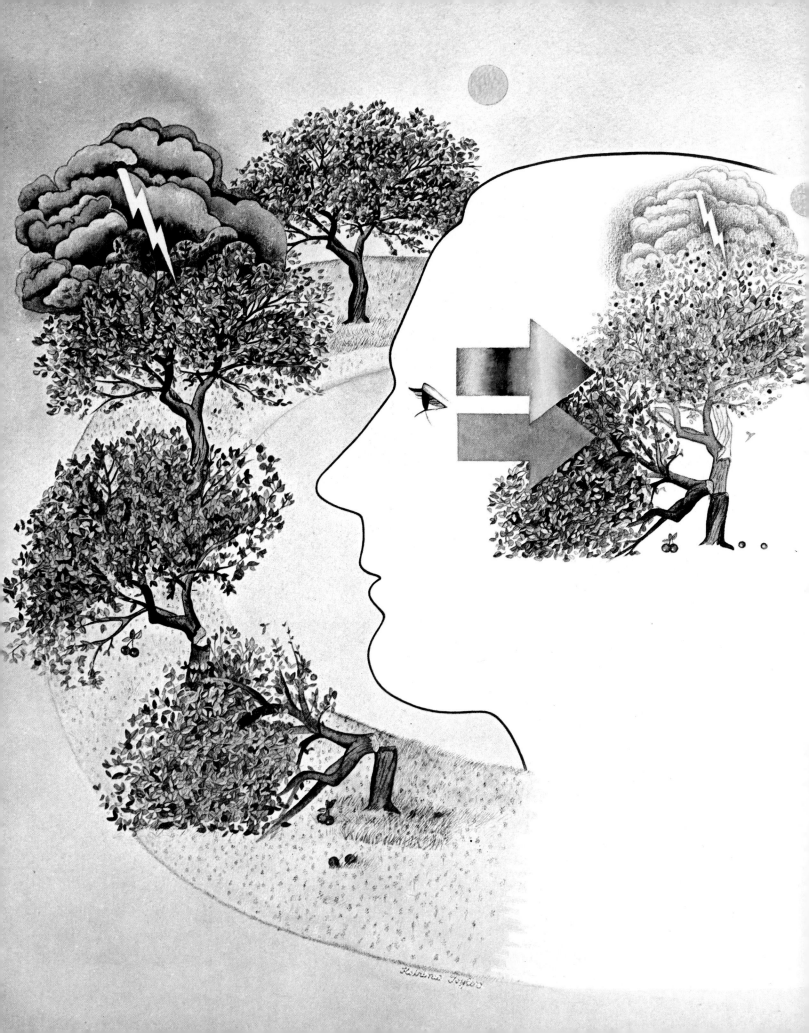

Sensory impulses entering the brain find accepting circuits or they fade away, according to immunologist Gerald Edelman. In theory, as the tree falls, the brain recycles related images within memory circuits.

When a foreign substance, or antigen, invades the body, the immune system produces a specific antibody to counteract it. The production of antibodies is a selective process. All of the information necessary to recognize antigens is already programmed in the system. When encountering an antigen, the system selects the antibody-producing cell most closely fitting the invading substance. The production of a specific antibody "leaves an imprint on the system that can serve as a 'memory' for a second encounter." Each encounter speeds the response as more cells are imprinted with the memory. According to Edelman, this amplification process is a critical part of making the system succeed.

Does a similar mechanism operate in the brain, Edelman asks, "and if so, at what level . . . cells, molecules or circuits of cells?" Edelman proposes that circuits consisting of 50 to 10,000 neurons serve as the basic processing units of the brain. The neurons are programmed from birth to form common code-recognizing groups.

Sensory signals entering the brain survey these code group circuits. Only those circuits which can read the incoming signal's code will respond. But just as we can understand a coded message before solving every letter, so the nerve circuits will respond to signals with codes they recognize but have not completely read. A memory of some type is created at the nerve synapse when the coded signal passes through, leaving behind its individual imprint. A quadrillion links between brain cells formed by neuron connections make up a network of brain circuits Edelman calls the "primary repertoire."

Many different circuits of the primary repertoire will recognize and respond to a signal entering the brain. The theorist believes this action strengthens the responding nerve circuits. The process prepares special groups of nerve cells that respond quickly when the same signal once again enters the system.

Through this selection process the group of primary circuits becomes transformed into a specialized "secondary repertoire." The secondary circuit group patterns itself to receive, amplify and retransmit the coded signals. Because individual experiences create unique variations in the primary repertoire, the secondary circuit patterns are distinct for every individual. No two human brains have the same neural circuits.

Edelman theorizes that the brain functions by a constant recycling of impulses among its many circuits. Initial sensory signals are received by groups called feature detectors or "recognizers" that are probably composed of physically related groups of circuits. After the signals are processed by the recognizers, other circuits called recognizers of recognizers (R of R) record the information in less specific forms. This information is then recycled, and picked up by other R of R groups or sent to parts of the brain controlling the body's actions.

He sees the brain "as a seething mass of patterns going on and off." New information from the senses activates recognizer circuits. Their reactions are recognized and recorded by R of R circuits. These processed signals then reenter the system and are read by other R of R groups as if they were external signals. This continual reexamining and comparing of recycled information with newly arriving sensory impulses may be what we call consciousness and self-awareness. It is a building process in each individual, suggests Edelman, whereby increasingly abstract patterns are stored in the R of R circuits. This may explain, he says, how man can adapt and respond to completely new information: "The most dramatic examples are the capabilities of some individuals to solve highly abstract problems in mathematics [or] generate new symbol structures of the complexity of a symphony."

His novel theory of brain organization has been supported by the work of his senior colleague, Vernon Mountcastle, chairman of Johns Hopkins University's department of physiology. According to Mountcastle, nerve cells within the brain group to form minicolumns, nearly 600 million of them. Minicolumns form, in turn, 600,000 larger structures he calls macrocolumns. These vertical columns can either process information separately or communicate with each other. Edelman believes that the columns may be the physical basis of the recognizer groups.

Another theory of brain organization utilizes the principles of holography, a photographiclike

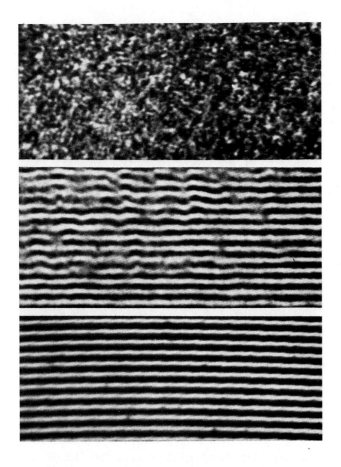

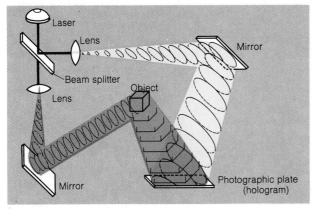

The surface of this holographic plate, at top, shows the image of interference patterns when enlarged 2,000 times. Split laser waves, at bottom, collide at the photo plate to record the holographic image.

process. To produce a hologram, the single wavelength light of a laser beam is split with a mirror. Half of the beam is aimed directly at the photographic plate; the other half bounces off the object to hit the plate. Instead of recording an image, the plate records interference patterns of the colliding light waves. To reconstruct the image, a laser is directed at the plate at the same angle as the original laser. The hologram appears as a three-dimensional image that can be turned and studied from different angles.

But the most remarkable aspect of holography remains on the plate. If a corner is broken off, it can be used to reconstruct the entire image. The image may be less distinct, but nonetheless complete. A single plate can record many different images if it is rotated so that the laser strikes at different angles. One cubic centimeter of the plate can hold ten billion bits of information. The only known system for storing information more sophisticated than the hologram is the brain.

The holographic theory developed from the unrelated studies of two men: Dennis Gabor, who won the Nobel Prize in 1971 for his discovery of holography; and neuropsychologist Karl Lashley, who, in the 1920s, first demonstrated that memory seems to be dispersed throughout the brain and not at specific points.

Lashley trained rats to run mazes and then removed various portions of their brains. He discovered that he could impair memory but not destroy it. Even when he cut major nerve pathways and removed as much as 90 percent of the visual cortex — the part of the brain that processes visual signals — his rats could still remember and perform complex activities.

Karl Pribram, a neurophysiologist at Stanford University, began his search for a model of brain function by drawing on Lashley's work. Pribram realized that the hologram was "unique as a storage device" because "every element in the original image is distributed over the entire photographic plate." He also found the holographic model "attractive because remembering or recollecting literally implies a reconstructive process." Pribram believes individual memories are encoded not in single neurons or pathways of neurons, but in a chemical pattern that causes

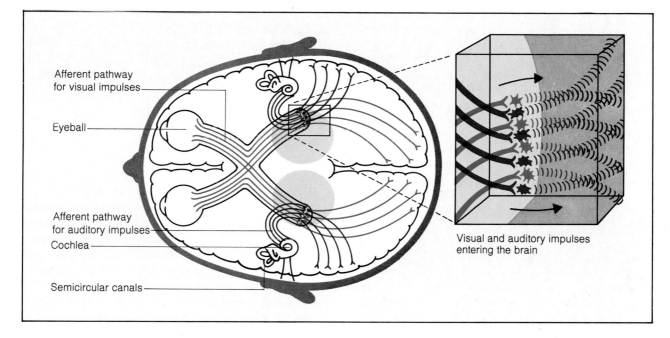

Afferent pathway
for visual impulses

Eyeball

Afferent pathway
for auditory impulses

Cochlea

Semicircular canals

Visual and auditory impulses
entering the brain

changes in trillions of synapses. Each synapse, therefore, may retain billions of memories.

Pribram believes that the three-dimensional hologram serves as a model for consciousness as well. The image that a person sees "is not on the photographic film. It's somewhere beyond; it's a projection. If the brain is holographically organized, conscious experience will be similarly projected when the right input comes in."

A brain organized holographically, in his view, should store information in a variety of ways. It could "read out the information in either linear or spatial fashion. The linear way is sequential, over time, and the spatial is simultaneous." He thinks that the holographic analogy accounts not only for our sensory perceptions such as vision and hearing, but also for the abstract perceptions of time and space. "Space and time are not in the brain," he says, "they are read out of it." His theory is so provocative that it has been used to explain psychic phenomena, spiritual experiences and even the structure of the universe.

Secrets of Brain Chemistry

While the brain's circuitry remains theoretical, scientists are rapidly revealing the secrets of its chemistry. In recent years, researchers have dis-

Pribram likens abstract thought processes to a hologram. Myriad impulses beam to the brain through the senses, converging and interfering as signals overlap within the brain's cells. The resulting impulses contain vast amounts of information forming memories that can be recalled at the same instant, individually or serially.

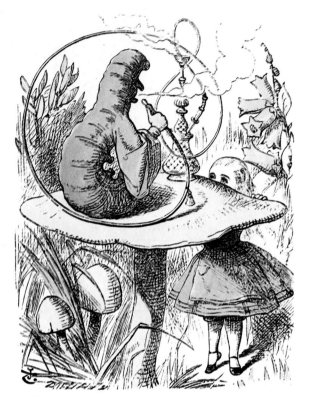

Puffing his opium pipe, a hookah, the caterpillar in Alice in Wonderland *demands of Alice, "Who are you?" For centuries, opium has been used to alter consciousness, to kill pain. Binding to opiate receptors on the neuron, the drug slows pain's passage from body to brain.*

covered nearly thirty chemicals that act as neurotransmitters, each designed to convey a different type of information. Some direct the activities of the glands and muscles; others regulate sleep and wakefulness or influence emotions and behavior. Perhaps the most exciting discovery may someday solve the mysteries of pain.

The key to the latest discoveries is opium, a powerful narcotic known to man at least since the days of the classical Greeks. For centuries it has been used in various forms to relieve pain and induce euphoria. The ability of opium to relieve pain is so great that it led one seventeenth-century physician to write: "Among the remedies which it has pleased Almighty God to give man to relieve his sufferings, none is so universal and so efficacious as opium." Unfortunately, as physicians subsequently discovered, opium and its derivatives — morphine, codeine and heroin — are addictive. They also produce severe mental and physical deterioration over time. One of the major goals of modern science has been to discover a nonaddictive opiate. In order to do so, however, scientists needed first to understand how opiates work to relieve pain and why they are addictive. In 1973, scientists at Johns Hopkins University found part of the answer.

Solomon H. Snyder and Candace Pert discovered that morphine and other opiates bind to specific sites, called opiate receptors, on the surface of nerve cells in the brain and spinal cord. Once locked to the receptors, the drug slows the rate at which the cell fires. Opiates relieve pain by reducing the number of signals traveling along pathways to the brain.

Snyder and his colleagues next began to map the location of opiate receptors in the brain. They found a dense band in the spinal cord, the first place where information about pain is processed. In the brain's medial thalamus, the seat of deep chronic pain, they discovered another thick region where opiates work efficiently.

"Why," Snyder wondered, "would nature put a receptor in our brain meant only to interact with the juice of a poppy?" The human body does not produce morphine, and it is unlikely that such specialized structures would exist without serving some normal function. Snyder and

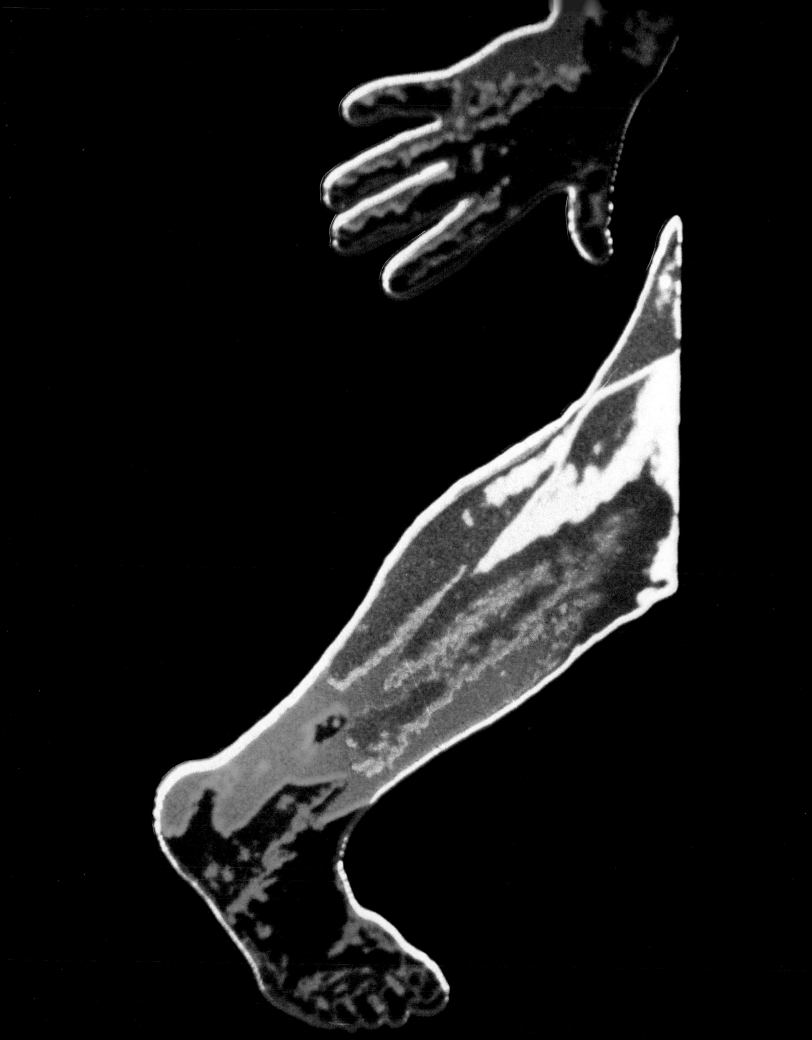

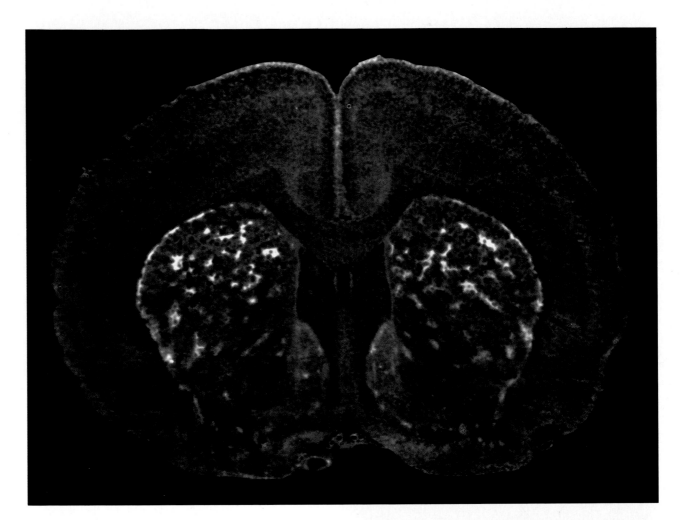

Opiate receptors fleck an autoradio-
graph of part of a rat's brain, above.
Special synaptic buttons, at right,
spray enkephalins into special receptors to slow the release of neurotransmitters in nearby nerve cells.
The reduced flow of impulses cuts
back waves of pain traveling to the
brain.

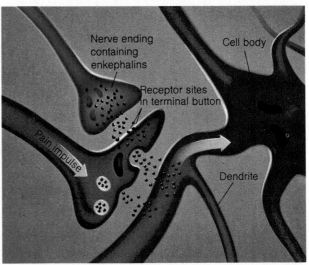

other scientists reasoned that opiate receptors must exist in order to interact with some substance already in the body. Teams of neuroscientists set out to find the proof.

In 1975, John Hughes and Hans Kosterlitz of the University of Aberdeen in Scotland isolated a brain chemical that acted on the opiate receptors. They named it enkephalin, meaning "in the head." A few months later Snyder and his colleagues reported the same discovery.

Both teams identified the substance as a peptide, or short chain of amino acids, the building blocks of proteins, and discovered that it occurs in two forms. Both of the enkephalin peptides consist of five amino acids, differing only in the last amino acid on the chain.

Enkephalins concentrate in nerve endings located near nerves containing opiate receptors. When a pain impulse enters the spinal cord, special neurons release the enkephalins. Fitting into a nearby nerve's opiate receptors, they suppress the release of neurotransmitters that would ordinarily pass along the pain signal and thereby lessen the feeling of pain.

Natural Painkillers

With the discovery of enkephalins, other pieces of the chemical puzzle began to fit together. In 1965, at the University of California in San Francisco, scientist C. H. Li had isolated a hormone, beta-lipotropin, from the pituitary gland near the base of the brain. Beta-lipotropin, a string of ninety-one amino acids, helps in the breakdown of fat. But he suspected there was more to it. Li discovered that one of the enkephalins was actually a portion of the hormone's amino acids.

Several research groups quickly focused on the pituitary in search of more opiate peptides. They did not find enkephalins in the pituitary, but they did find substances acting like opiates and containing the enkephalin's amino acid sequence. Most of the opiatelike activity in the pituitary seems to come from a chain of thirty-one amino acids called beta-endorphin. The role of beta-endorphin, however, is still unknown.

Enkephalins in the brain seem to be unrelated in origin to endorphins in the pituitary, although endorphins contain the same sequence of five amino acids. Researchers found that beta-lipotropin is itself part of a larger chain known as ACTH, a stress-related hormone released when a person experiences pain. This hormone and endorphin might work together to help the body handle great pain. The large molecule, scientists suggest, could break into its smaller pieces to handle specific targets.

About two dozen more peptides appear to be neurotransmitters with opiate characteristics. The study of enkephalins and related chemicals has led scientists to speculate that the body possesses a special chemical control system to cope with pain and stress. They theorize that many people seem indifferent to pain under stress because of the body's ability to call forth additional supplies of these natural painkillers.

Enkephalin research has also helped explain the chemistry of narcotic addiction. Under normal circumstances, scientists believe, enkephalins occupy a certain number of opiate receptors. Morphine relieves pain by occupying receptors that are left unfilled. Too much morphine may cause a cutoff of enkephalin production, leaving receptors open. The body then craves more morphine to fill the unoccupied receptors and to cut down the pain. If denied morphine, all of the opiate receptors remain empty, causing painful withdrawal symptoms.

Enkephalins may also regulate mood. These chemicals are heavily concentrated in the limbic system, the area of the brain involved in regulating emotion. Enkephalins in this region may act as the body's own "natural high" to counteract disappointment and prevent depression. The euphoria produced by morphine and other opiates lends support to this theory, but the actual process by which enkephalins influence mood is not yet known.

Scientists believe that research into the body's natural opiates may lead to the development of nonaddictive painkillers and, ultimately, to a complete understanding of the complex chemistry of pain. Their predictions have been optimistic but restrained. "So far, we have only looked at perhaps 40 percent of the neurons in the human brain," notes Candace Pert. "I'd like to know a little more about the other 60 percent."

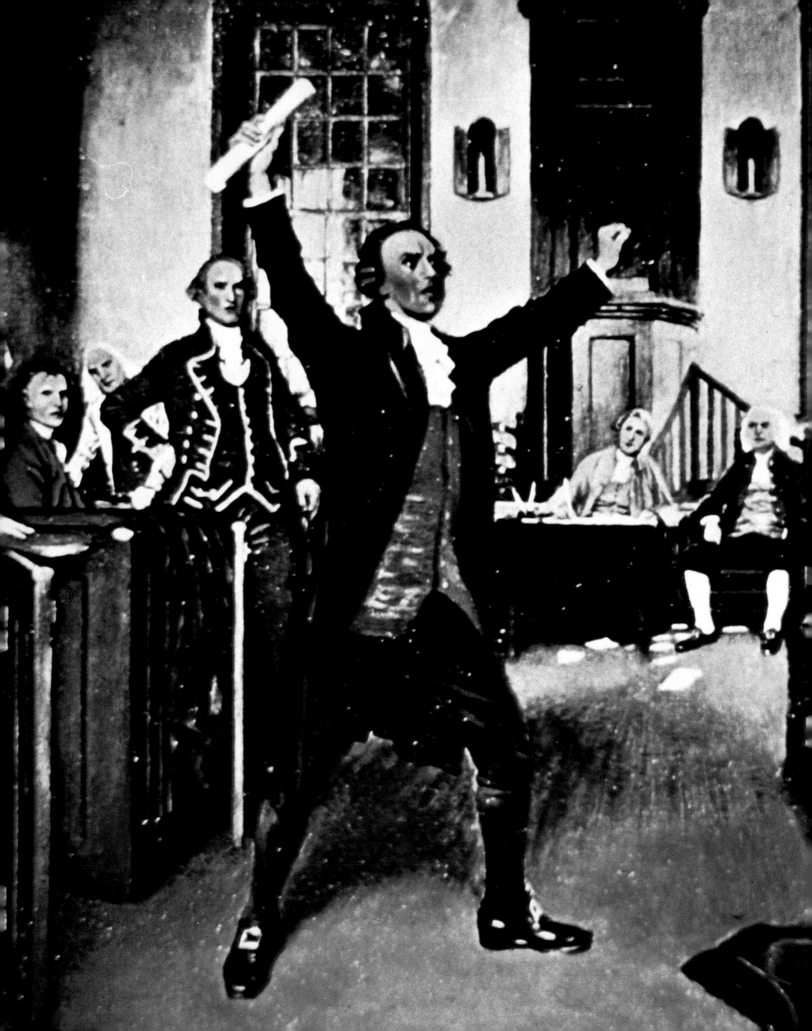

Chapter 4

The Gift of Language

*"Give me liberty or give me death,"
thundered Patrick Henry at the
Virginia Convention convened at St.
John's Episcopal Church in
Richmond, Virginia, 1775. His
words shook the American colonies,
triggering a clamor for independence
that exploded in revolution. The
power of speech, moving men and
nations as no other force, uniquely
sets humans apart from animals.
Yet, the origins of language remain
one of the brain's most baffling
mysteries.*

anguage is the light of the mind," wrote English philosopher John Stuart Mill. With language, the conscious self shines forth; it enables us to turn our awareness outward, to share our humanity, our rationality and our creativity. Philosopher Karl Popper believes that with the emergence of articulate man came "the world of the products of the human mind, a world of myths, of fairy tales . . . of poetry."

The production of speech is finely organized. Air we breathe is abruptly converted by the valve action of the larynx into the sound waves of speech. Vocal cords release air in short bursts, making sound waves by breaking the air into minute, oscillating puffs having a regular pitch. The brain refines these sound waves into acoustical patterns that make intelligible not only the thrust of our meaning — a question or command, an accusation or plea — but its emotional content as well. The sudden surge of sound flows through the double-story vocal tract of nose and mouth. Masses of brain-controlled muscle and tissue mold and alter the shape of the tract walls. They cause the soft palate to lift, shutting off air to the nose. They prompt the tongue to change shape and position, the lips to purse or spread, channeling the air to crash against, roar over or hiss between the teeth.

The brain is also specialized for speech. Two of its three language centers were named for the nineteenth-century scientists who discovered them. Wernicke's area, in the left temporal lobe, enables us to comprehend speech. Broca's area, in the folds of the same lobe, lies next to the brain area that coordinates movement of the tongue, lips, palate and vocal cords. Broca's area controls the flow of words from brain to mouth. Every minute, two hundred syllables are exquisitely synchronized in what experimental phoneticist Dennis Fry calls "the most brilliant technical achievement of the human brain."

"Say cheese," calls the camera-man — and the word forms signals in the hearer's primary auditory area, at right. Wernicke's area structures the signals, passing its program via the arcuate fasciculus, the nerve pathway to Broca's area, which directs the motor area to make the mouth say "cheese." If written, the word begins in the visual cortex, below; the angular gyrus must then trigger in Wernicke's area an auditory form of "cheese."

THE HEARD WORD

Arcuate fasciculus

Motor area

Primary auditory area

Broca's area

Wernicke's area

THE WRITTEN WORD

Arcuate fasciculus

Motor area

Angular gyrus

Broca's area

Wernicke's area

Primary visual area

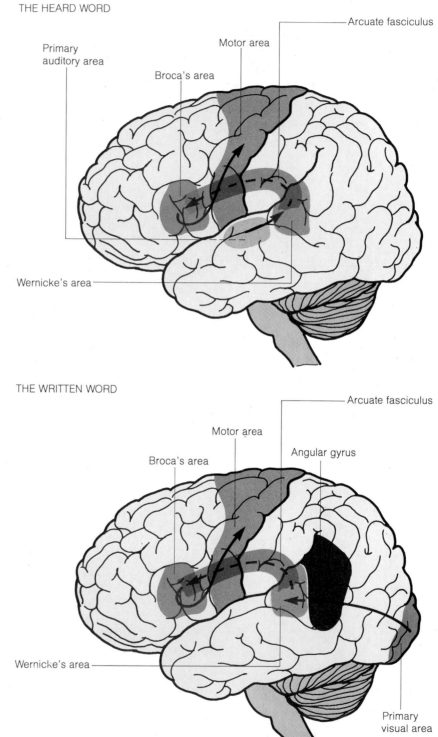

Pierre Paul Broca

Mapping the Articulate Brain

On a dusty shelf in the basement of the École de Médecine in Paris, a bottled brain rests in murky fluid. The wooden block supporting the jar bears the label "Brain of a man Leborgne called Tan aphasic."

In the spring of 1861, Tan, a terminally ill fifty-one-year-old man, came under the care of surgeon Pierre Paul Broca. For twenty-one years, an unknown affliction had stripped almost all but the meaningless utterance "tan, tan" from his vocabulary. He understood what was said to him and communicated by using facial expressions and hand gestures.

Tan's case sparked more than the usual curiosity. The Société d'Anthropologie, an organization founded by Broca two years earlier, had held heated discussions on the relationship between language and the brain. Broca, differing with most scientists of the day, argued that language ability must be located in one region of the brain. Realizing that Tan could help prove his theory, Broca gently tested the sick man, recording his powers and his disabilities.

One week later, Tan died. At the meeting of the Société the next day, Broca, with his proud father listening from the audience, presented his findings of the autopsy. Areas of

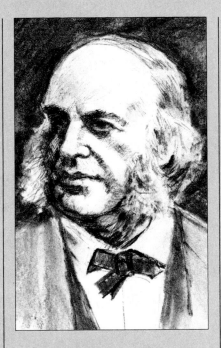

the brain appeared to be recently softened, probably contributing to Tan's late disabilities, which included the loss of mental keenness and paralysis. But the oldest lesion, thought Broca, seemed to be a region of Tan's left cerebral hemisphere where a piece of tissue as big as a hen's egg was missing. Broca reasoned that the oldest damage would correspond with Tan's earliest symptom. "Therefore," he concluded, "everything points to the fact that . . . the lesion of the frontal lobe was the cause of the loss of speech."

His conclusion was built on simple observation but the

implications were anything but simple. Broca's remarkable study of an unfortunate man removed the powers of language from the lofty mind and traced them to the firm roots of the physical brain. It was a scientific milestone.

Broca's conclusion shook the Société. Debate intensified as a whirlwind of religious and political questions arose. The young surgeon remained cool, however, taking care not to overestimate his revolutionary findings. Even when, several months later, a patient with a similar language impairment proved to have a lesion in the exact same spot of the brain, Broca remarked, "I am . . . disposed to attribute to pure coincidence the absolute identity of the site of the lesions in my two patients." And after studying the brains of fifteen such patients, all with similar lesions, Broca said, "but all this is too hypothetical; we must await further facts."

For all his caution, it is evident that Broca sensed the significance of his findings. Unlike other brains he had studied, Broca did not dissect Tan's brain; after showing it to the Société, he preserved it for placement in a museum. Almost forgotten, it remains in Paris today, mute evidence of the articulate brain.

When words are heard, the sounds pass to the auditory area of the cortex, flashing from there in neurological codes to the adjacent Wernicke's area, where they are unscrambled into understandable patterns of words. If the words are repeated aloud, the patterns must shift forward from Wernicke's area along a bundle of linking nerve fibers to Broca's area. Once here, they arouse the nearby motor area controlling the movement of speech muscles.

"Language frees us to a large extent from . . . the senses," wrote psychologist H. L. Teuber. "It provides a tool for representing absent objects and for manipulating them hypothetically in 'one's mind.'" It would seem essential to the production of language, said Teuber, that there be some brain mechanism for linking the senses, "for identifying an object felt with an object seen, and both with the object we can name." This appears to be the task of the third language center, the angular gyrus, a structure lying behind Wernicke's area in the midst of the brain regions receiving sensory signals. The angular gyrus bridges the gap between the speech we hear and the language we read and write. It transforms speech sounds into the visual messages needed to write what we hear and converts visual messages from reading into the sound patterns required to recite poetry from a book.

Language Gone Awry

But researchers do not know which parts of the brain produce original, unprompted speech. Neuroscientists believe vocabulary is stored in many parts of the brain, each connected to the language centers, because wherever there is brain damage there is usually a naming disorder.

Brain damage to the language centers produces aphasia, creating distinctive, abnormal speech. Patients with damage to Wernicke's area suffer receptive aphasia, making their language meaningless, even though the words carry a normal rhythm. A patient, asked his profession, replied, "Me? Yes sir. I'm a male demaploze on my own. I still know my tubaboys what for I have that's gone hell and some of them go."

When damage is confined to Broca's area, a person is literally at a loss for words. Broca's

aphasiacs speak in a characteristic telegraphic manner, as though some words remain trapped inside the brain while a few others squeeze through. Asked why he was in the hospital after suffering a stroke, one patient said, "Arm no good. . . . Speech . . . can't say . . . talk, you see."

When the connection between Broca's and Wernicke's areas is damaged, the patient may understand other people and produce meaningful thoughts. But the thoughts are expressed in language as meaningless as the language produced by Wernicke's aphasia. If the angular gyrus is damaged, a person may be able to repeat the words he hears but not those he reads.

Programmed for Dominance

More evidence that the brain is specialized for language comes from tests showing that ninety-seven of every hundred patients with language disorders have suffered damage in the left hemisphere. But scientists caution against concluding that language is confined exclusively to the left half of the brain.

Neuroscientists think that children under the age of ten or until puberty have a capacity to develop language in both hemispheres of the brain. If a child suffers injury to the left hemisphere's language centers, the earlier the injury the greater his chance of recovering language skills. The right hemisphere takes over, compensating for the loss. It is a phenomenon not easily explained, but psychologist Charles Furst suggests, "There is a great deal of plasticity in brain organization among children which . . . seems to decrease dramatically at about age fourteen." Furst also thinks that changes in brain organization may go on throughout life: "Perhaps we continue to rearrange our neural furniture to accommodate changing . . . needs."

Neurologist Norman Geschwind warns against overemphasizing the rigidity of linguistic assignments to specific sites. Instances of recovery from language disorders suggest to him that the brain is endowed with alternative stores of learning in the opposite brain hemisphere that remain dormant unless the dominant left half is injured.

An early struggle for linguistic dominance between the hemispheres may be implicated in one

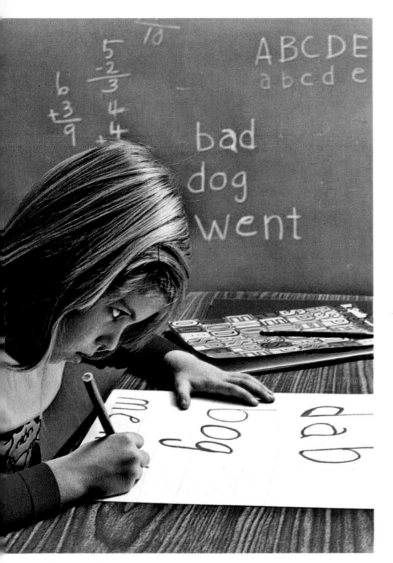

The eye sees bad *but the hand writes* dab *in the language disorder dyslexia. Language centers in the brain's left hemisphere seem to have backup systems in the right; when neither dominates, dyslexia results.*

grave language defect called alexia or, more commonly, dyslexia. In dyslexia, otherwise normal children may read words from right to left, mix up letters like *p* and *q*, read upside down and write backwards with either hand. Dyslexia is believed to result from the failure of one hemisphere of the brain to seize the faculty of language. Both hemispheres may then try to speak or read, with the attendant dyslexic errors.

Using a novel test developed by Juhn Wada of the University of British Columbia in Vancouver, Canada, researchers can determine which hemisphere controls speech, or if both halves vie for language supremacy. In the Wada test, the fast-acting anesthetic sodium amytal is injected into the neck's carotid arteries, major arteries feeding the brain. To verify left hemisphere dominance, the patient is instructed to count aloud; he stops counting when the anesthetic reaches the controlling hemisphere of the brain.

In clinical studies on stammering, researchers used the Wada test. They first injected the left carotid artery. After the injection, the patients began to count, hesitated and continued. The test, repeated on the right side, produced the same results. Like dyslexia, stammering seems to indicate competing hemispheres.

When does the left hemisphere begin to develop its language centers? Experts generally agree with Canadian psychologist Donald Hebb that no simple theory of learning can account for the phenomenon of language, but certain benchmarks in its growth appear in every culture: "It seems certain that the baby is born with a special sensitivity . . . to patterns of sound in human speech, and with special equipment . . . for the understanding, organization and production of speech. But this equipment, to become functional, may still require the effects of experience." By the age of five most children have completed the basic language acquisition process, hurdling the obstacles of grammar in stages.

During the first six months of life, the babbling of most babies sounds the same. Very soon thereafter, the child begins to learn his native tongue by experimenting with and imitating the fundamental sounds he hears. These basic sounds, or phonemes, differ in number and vari-

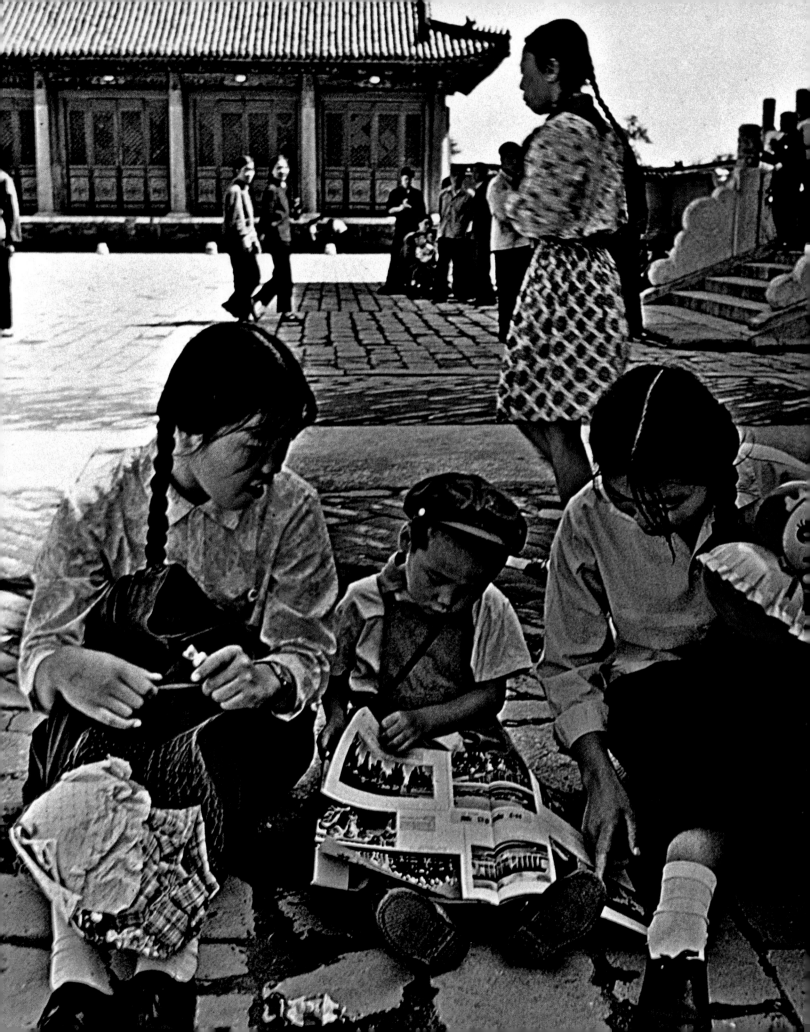

ation according to the language. The English-speaking baby may burble "th," one of forty-five phonemes, while some babies in the Soviet Union begin to voice the first of seventy-one phonemes. Within a year, the baby strings a number of them together to form morphemes, the smallest meaningful words or word elements — single-syllable words like *man* and units such as *ly* in the word *manly*.

Between the ages of one and two, the child combines words to produce meaningful sentences. Two-year-old children have a vocabulary ranging from 300 to 600 words. Infants put sentences together without prepositions, articles and pronouns; their language forms are simple. In the two-word stage, the child typically uses a subject with a verb: (Daddy go), or a verb with an object: (Bring it). The beginner also forms possessives by saying "Mommy dress" and indicates action, declaring "Drink milk." Struggling with the concept of time, children use the present tense before trying to grasp the past tense. The more abstract future is acquired even later. Children place the negatives "no" and "not" at the beginning or end of a sentence. They learn to refine the use of pronouns by substitution: from "I didn't do something" to "I didn't do anything."

The speed with which children fashion correct grammar is no measure of intelligence. Like sculptors shaping clay, children master language through practice, even in private monologues. Researcher Ruth Weir of Stanford University taped her son's verbal ramblings with a recorder hidden in his bedroom: "What color . . . what color blanket . . . what color mop . . . what color glass . . . what color TV . . . red ant . . . fire . . . like lipstick . . . blanket . . . now the blue blanket . . . what color TV . . . what color horse . . . then what color table . . . then what color fire . . . here yellow spoon."

The blissful ignorance of youth provides its own confidence. Harvard University professor Courtney Cazden suggests children take less heed of frequent adult correction than they do of their own trial and error. The word *why* is repeatedly posed not to get information but to keep the conversation going so that the child can practice the forms of social dialogue. By the time the

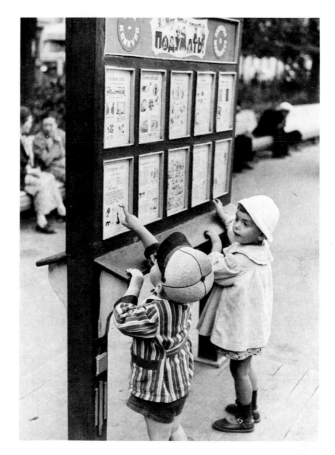

child is six or seven, changes in grammar may be extremely subtle; the polishing process continues at least until the age of ten.

Language Universals

Just how children absorb the complexities of language defies agreement among the experts. Psycholinguist Noam Chomsky of M.I.T. theorizes that "very deep and restrictive principles that determine the nature of human language . . . are rooted in . . . the human mind." These principles account for the creative aspect of language, enabling human beings to continually compose new sentences instead of repeating a fixed number of phrases.

According to Chomsky, the human brain is genetically programmed for language development. He thinks children learn language in the sense that maturing parts of the brain enable them to recognize basic regularities in the speech they

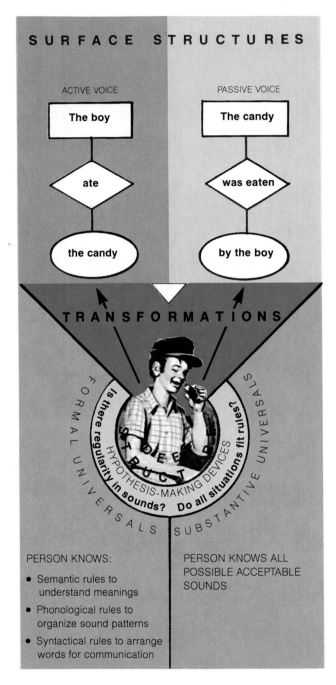

SURFACE STRUCTURES

ACTIVE VOICE

The boy

ate

the candy

PASSIVE VOICE

The candy

was eaten

by the boy

TRANSFORMATIONS

FORMAL UNIVERSALS

Is there regularity in sounds?

HYPOTHESIS-MAKING DEVICES

Do all situations fit rules?

DEEP STRUCTURE

SUBSTANTIVE UNIVERSALS

PERSON KNOWS:

- Semantic rules to understand meanings
- Phonological rules to organize sound patterns
- Syntactical rules to arrange words for communication

PERSON KNOWS ALL POSSIBLE ACCEPTABLE SOUNDS

All humans are born with language universals, believes psycholinguist Noam Chomsky. Deep structures containing ideas transform thoughts into different sentence structures without losing the meaning.

hear around them. These regularities, or language universals, says Chomsky, take two basic forms, substantive and formal.

Substantive universals are the sounds of speech. Thus a child would recognize the sounds of *b*, *p* or *q* as parts of speech but would reject the sound of a cough or a hiccup. Most linguists agree with this idea. Chomsky's concept of formal universals is more complicated and controversial: he believes children instinctively know how the grammar of a language should be organized. Humans have an internal set of rules, says Chomsky, enabling them to recognize the "deep structure" of a sentence. No matter which way a sentence is phrased — Bill gave Linda a dime, Linda was given a dime by Bill, a dime was given to Linda by Bill — the same meaning is expressed and understood even though the structure of the sentence changes.

The late Swiss psychologist Jean Piaget, a pioneer in the study of child thought and language, opposed Chomsky's theory of language acquisition. While acknowledging the existence of something resembling deep structures, Piaget argued that they were not genetically programmed. Instead, he believed, children acquire language by stages. Each stage carries its own set of grammatical rules from which children construct more mature stages with new sets of rules.

Scientists differ over whether language is innate, but they agree that expecting a child to learn a language without the experience of talking to others is like trying to start a car without switching on the ignition. According to psycholinguist Breyne Arlene Moskowitz, "Many of the severe language abnormalities found in children can in some way be traced to interruptions of the normal acquisition process." An asthmatic boy, confined to home and reared by deaf parents, neither understood nor spoke by the age of three, even though he was exposed daily to television. Moskowitz believes it is the process of dialogue that enables the child to develop language.

But is there an age beyond which a child cannot acquire a language? Eric Lenneberg of the Harvard Medical School suggested that "puberty marks a milestone . . . for the facility of language acquisition." He drew on circumstantial evidence

Noam Chomsky

Bold Voice of Linguistics

Noam Chomsky's approach to the study of language is so strikingly different from traditional theories that his ideas about the nature and structure of language have been dubbed "the Chomskyan Revolution." Almost singlehandedly, he has dramatically reshaped the modern study of linguistics.

When Chomsky first entered linguistics in the late 1940s, the field was dominated by taxonomists who classified bits and pieces of language much as a botanist would classify plants. Chomsky felt that classification by form or behavior was not an adequate method of studying language. To investigate language only on its surface, he argued, was to ignore its complexities: We "lose sight of the need for explanation when phenomena are too familiar and 'obvious.'" The direction of Chomsky's studies reignited the classic debate between rationalism and empiricism.

In the early seventeenth century, French philosopher René Descartes refurbished the rationalist view of the structure of the human mind. His theory, called Cartesian, held the belief that man had innate ideas which gave order to the mind and provided a structure for learning. The opposing point of view, empiricism,

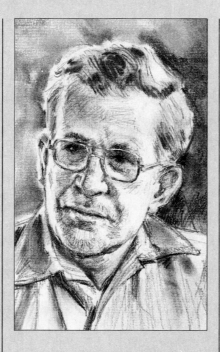

strengthened some fifty years later by the English philosopher John Locke, held that the mind was a blank tablet — a *tabula rasa* — to be filled in by experience. "No man's knowledge," argued Locke, "can go beyond experience."

Three hundred years later, this debate wedged itself into linguistics, the Lockean position championed by behavioral psychologist B. F. Skinner. Behaviorism is a modern application of empiricist thought and Skinner, its most influential supporter. Skinner calls language "verbal behavior," learned like any other behavior. In essence, he believes that

a child gradually learns to speak by repeating what he hears and receiving reinforcement in the form of praise from parents.

Chomsky, on the other hand, argues that language use is too complex and creative, the laws of grammar too intricate, to be absorbed by mere repetition. Cartesian-inspired, his theories are based on the idea that man possesses innate, universal brain structures for language acquisition. "Empiricist and later behaviorist psychology are firmly grounded in the doctrine that there is no nontrivial theory of human nature," Chomsky scoffs in *Reflections on Language.*

Chomsky's field, psycholinguistics, is a blend of psychology, linguistics and philosophy that aims to understand, through language, the workings of the human mind. Now as well-established as the behavioral interpretation of language, psycholinguistics ensures no end to the debate. "It may be beyond the limits of human intelligence," Chomsky once observed, "to understand how human intelligence works." But Noam Chomsky is not a pessimist; if, as he believes, language is a mirror of the mind, then Chomsky is first in line at the looking glass.

of the physical and biochemical development of the brain, adding that when "language acquisition comes to be inhibited, the brain can also be shown to have reached its mature state."

Linguistics professor Susan Curtiss of UCLA cites a number of important chemical processes that determine the maturity of the brain at the age of about ten. "After this critical period only a small amount of language can be acquired," she proposes, "and even this cannot be acquired in the normal fashion, or to the same degree. Vocabulary can be acquired but syntax, especially, cannot be acquired past this point."

Curtiss's theory is based on a decade of studying a girl named Genie. Admitted to a hospital in 1970, Genie was nearly fourteen years old and unable to speak a word. From the age of about twenty months, she had been isolated by her parents in a small, closed room. She could not stand erect and uttered only a throaty whimper.

Genie quickly responded to speech and imitated single words. Within two years, she learned some basic grammatical structures and used a vocabulary of hundreds of words. But ten years after hospitalization, Curtiss observes, Genie's language "is still very impaired by impoverished grammar." Her speech is high-pitched, breathy, and intelligible only to those who know her well.

She must have passed the years, think those who work with her, "absorbing every visual stimulus, every crack in the paint, every nuance of color and form," thereby stimulating the right hemisphere of her brain into normal development. Tests suggest to researchers that Genie's right hemisphere does all the work of language in addition to all other cognitive functions. "This makes her unique," says Curtiss, "because she has one hemisphere doing these things in the presence of an intact left hemisphere."

The Ape Controversy

As Genie confounds the experts, other researchers are sparring with the conventional wisdom which reserves to humans the gift of language. Chomsky ridicules the notion that mankind's closest relatives, the chimpanzees, can ever be candidates for human dialogue: "It's about as likely that an ape will prove to have a language ability as that there is an island somewhere with a species of flightless birds waiting for human beings to teach them to fly."

Chimpanzees were bequeathed the handicap of anatomical differences. Stanford University anthropologist Suzanne Chevalier-Skolnikoff cites the primates' vocal chambers as part of the reason apes cannot, or do not learn to talk. Within a few months after birth the human baby's tongue and larynx move from a forward to a downward position in the throat, creating a natural passage for easy breathing and the sounds of speech. By contrast, the tongue and larynx of the chimpanzee remain in the forward position. Man enjoys additional advantages of a nimbler tongue, more flexible lips and a lighter jawbone to form words. Many scientists also suspect there may be elusive neurological distinctions vital for speech.

But even if they can't speak, can apes understand the meaning of language? Paleontologist Adrian Desmond, author of *The Ape's Reflexion*, believes that "linguists have a prejudice toward the auditory as the only mode in which language can be expressed." Researchers argue whether apes can learn a gestural form of language.

Psychologists Allen and Beatrice Gardner of the University of Nevada tried to teach their chimp, Washoe, the American Sign Language of the deaf, ASL. They taught Washoe more than 240 signs for nouns, adjectives and verbs. The Gardners reported that Washoe put together words after learning her first eight signs. They speculate she may even have developed poetic license by signaling the signs for "water bird" when she saw a swan gliding in water. The psychologists insist that Washoe invented meaningful combinations of words, such as "cry hurt food" after eating a piquant radish.

David Premack, professor of psychology at the University of California at Santa Barbara, used plastic-covered metal shapes and a magnetic slate to teach his chimp, Sarah, more than 130 words. Initially placing fruit next to a shape, Premack removed the fruit and gave it to Sarah only after she placed the shape on the language board.

Columbia University psychologist Herbert Terrace playfully named a two-week-old chimp Nim Chimsky and coached him to learn 125

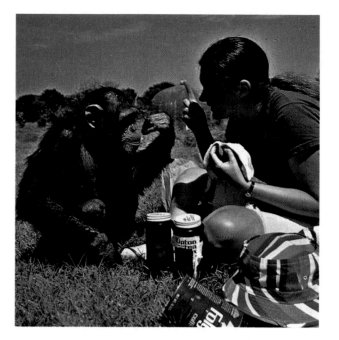

Aping its instructor, a chimpanzee learns to converse — not in speech ill suited to its vocal apparatus, but in sign language. Many scientists say such apes are using language; simian brains may include a primitive counterpart to human language centers. Others see only elaborate conditioning used to win rewards — brainy behavior, but not language.

ASL signs. But after four years of tutoring and studying 5,200 combinations of Nim's signs in search of structural regularities, Terrace concluded that the chimp's sequences lacked "the syntactic structure of sentences." Terrace reached his decision after examining video tapes of Nim and other chimps. "The closer I looked, the more I regarded the many reported instances of language as elaborate tricks for obtaining reward," he wrote. Terrace suggests that the apes rely heavily on prompting. He dismisses Washoe's "water bird," believing that the sign she made was probably a juxtaposition of objects named separately rather than a deliberate description of something she had never seen before.

But Premack accuses those who reject ape language of "a certain amount of scrambling to protect the uniqueness of man." He assesses his own tests ambivalently: "It could indicate an incapacity of the species, or merely that the training was improper." Steven Rose, one of the founders of the British Brain Research Association, muses, "Perhaps chimpanzees, too, have 'naming centers'? The human capacity for speech is certainly unique. But the gulf between it and the behavior of animals no longer seems unbridgeable."

Intelligent Machines

At the other end of the spectrum are the scientists attempting to program computers to formulate language. To Moskowitz the task is formidable: "Ten linguists working full time for ten years to analyze the structure of the English language could not program a computer with the ability for language acquired by an average child in the first ten or even five years of life."

Undaunted, Roger Schank, chairman of the computer science department at Yale University, analyzes words for their meaning before programming them into the computer. In the sentence "John prevented Mary from leaving the room by locking the door," Schank programs the computer to understand that the word *prevent* signifies a relationship between events: John locked the door to prevent Mary from leaving the room.

Schank programs his computers to make inferences. He studies why people talk to each other, how they select what they want to say, to what

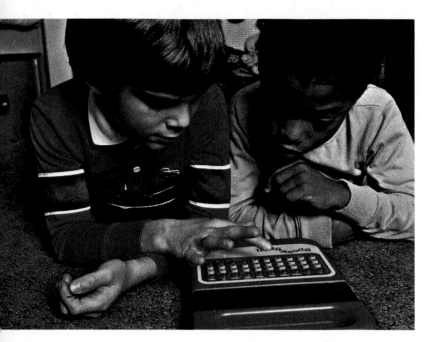

A brain in a box helps two young human brains absorb the rudiments of spelling. Within its limited vocabulary, it never fails — unless its batteries do. Yet not even the brainiest computers can challenge the skill of these youngsters in the use of words to communicate.

extent situations define what should be said and precisely what should be said at any given time. "In natural language processing," Schank believes that "conversation is probably the most important aspect under study."

The computers make inferences from what he calls everyday scripts. The phrase "I flew in a plane," he says, "carries the inference that I packed my bags, drove to the airport, waited in line, bought a ticket and then boarded the plane." Computer scientists at Yale have developed a computer called SAM (Script Applier Mechanism) which summarizes stories. Fed with a thirty-nine-word story, SAM can quickly deliver a seventeen-word summary of salient facts.

To what extent can these so-called intelligent machines understand the depth and nuance of human feeling hidden in language? Computer scientist Joseph Weizenbaum of M.I.T. contends that there are human experiences, such as love, which the computer cannot share.

Schank gives qualified approval. "I'm inclined to agree with him if he is talking of the true empathy, the real understanding in love. But a lot of the complexities in people can be modeled in the machines. We have built programs to simulate memory and ability, to respond to the same rules in certain situations. A computer can compose poetry, though I wouldn't guarantee it would be very good. But it is certainly not out of bounds. We have programs in which the computer tells stories. And we can program what dating is like and the desire to fall in love. But if you ask whether the computer will cry, the answer is no."

Schank's team at the Artificial Intelligence Project has programmed computers with knowledge about the aims and political stances of individuals. According to Schank the computers are then able to understand actions and motives behind goals, and also to differentiate between right- and left-wing political attitudes.

But no computer can initiate conversation. As language theoretician Eric Lenneberg saw it, a sentence is somewhat analagous to a mosaic, "put together stone after stone, yet the picture as a whole must have come into being in the artist's mind before he began to lay down the pieces." To date this is a faculty only humans possess.

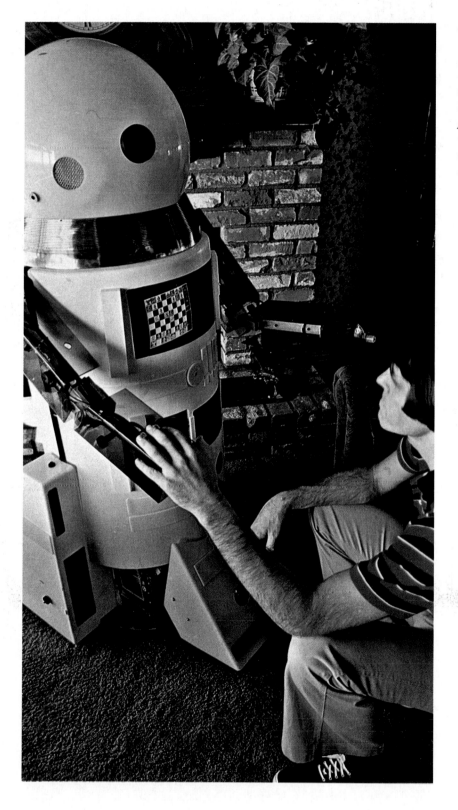

Einstein of robots, a computerized wonder named ARGON pauses in its varied tasks to match wits with a human at chess. Smart money bets on the human, though in weighing his moves his brain completes only four or five operations per second. Computers can complete several million — yet none has consistently checkmated a chess master.

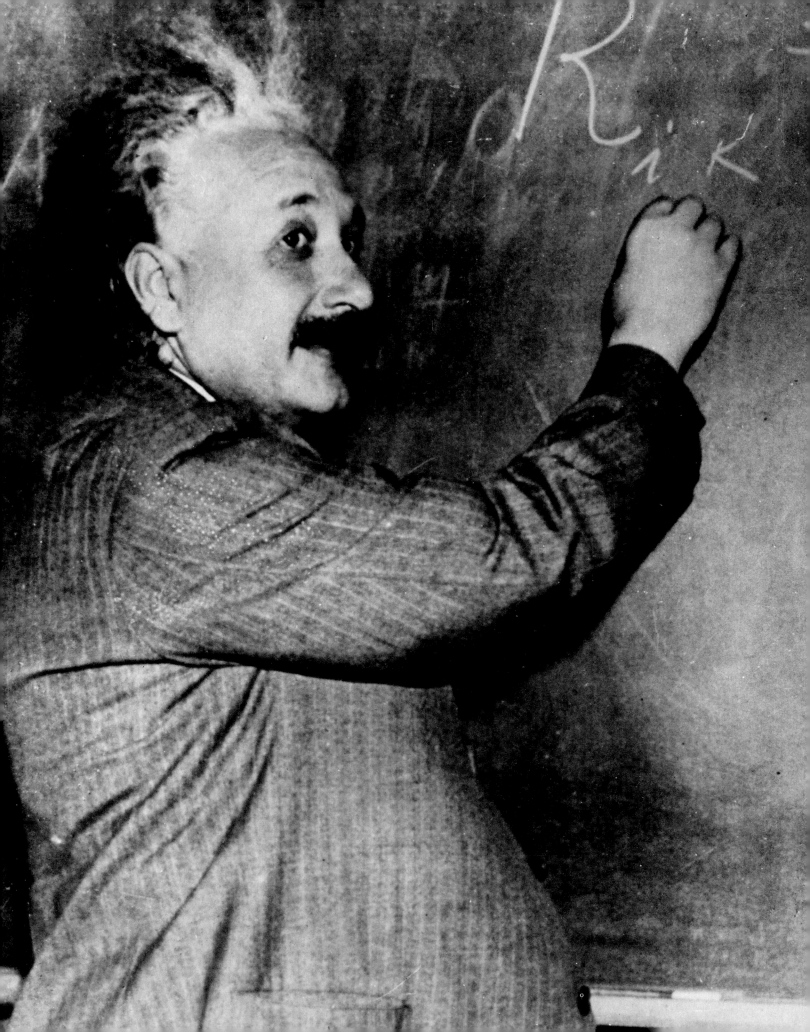

Chapter 5

Intelligence and Creativity

"Intelligence is what intelligence tests test," concluded psychologist Edwin Boring in 1923. If his ironic definition of intelligence seems like defining electricity as "what makes a light bulb glow," the comparison is appropriate. Both intelligence and electricity lack complete explanations that appeal to our common sense. Yet in the presence of either, we recognize the undeniable fact of their existence. Intelligence, however, is not as precisely measurable as a sustained surge of electric current, and intelligence tests do not enjoy the matter-of-fact acceptance society accords the light bulb. Just what are the ingredients of the cerebral recipe? This still unanswered question and the problem of measuring something not easily defined have led to the durability of Boring's unilluminating definition.

Despite the absence of a meaningful definition, something is there at work, enabling us, in the words of psychologist David Weschler, "to act purposefully, to think rationally, and to deal effectively with [the] environment." This force may be deliberate, logical and predictable or disordered, intuitive and spontaneous. It allows us to solve problems step by step or in a single burst of insight, to think in images or symbols and to take ideas apart, putting them back together in unique ways. In short, it is something exhibiting all the mental abilities that make mankind the highest order of mammal.

Gauging Intelligence

Nearly a hundred years ago, Sir Francis Galton, a nineteenth-century English mathematician and half-cousin of Charles Darwin, made the first scientific investigations into the nature of intelligence. Galton believed that intelligence was based on the keenness of the senses. He reasoned that since we gather information through our senses, intelligence should vary according to the sharpness of our perceptual abilities. Testing his

"I want to know how God created this world," wrote Albert Einstein, scientist, humanist, seeker of large truths. The universe his blackboard, Einstein changed the world — its concepts, its course — and so proved man's mind a most potent tool.

Verbal, mathematical and reasoning aptitudes are expressions of intelligence that lend themselves to current standardized tests. Other skills and talents, however, defy such precise measurement.

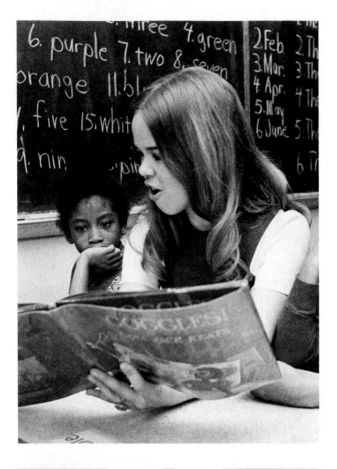

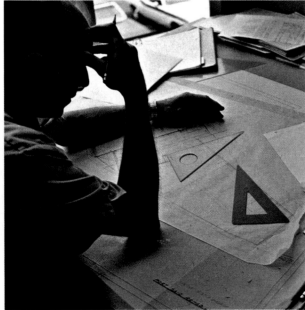

theory at the London Exhibition of 1884, Sir Francis measured the eyesight, hearing, reaction time and other perceptual-motor skills of more than 9,000 visitors. Galton was disappointed to discover that there was little relationship between perceptual abilities and intellectual achievement. Ordinary citizens frequently tested higher than distinguished British scientists.

Around the turn of the twentieth century, French psychologist Alfred Binet, the father of modern intelligence testing, argued that reasoning, judgment, comprehension and the capacity for self-criticism, rather than keenness of the senses, were "the essential activities of intelligence." At the request of the French government, Binet designed a test to predict whether a child would succeed in the standard school or require a special program of study. Designed to sort schoolchildren by their mental abilities, Binet's tests included identifying familiar objects, finding rhymes for a given word and repeating lists of numbers. Binet discovered that brighter children performed at a mental age more advanced than their chronological age, while duller children performed below. In 1912, German psychologist William Stern suggested an intelligence quotient, or IQ, could be computed by dividing a child's mental age by his chronological age and multiplying that number by one hundred.

The success of Binet's test in predicting academic performance ignited an explosion of aptitude, achievement and personality tests. In 1914, the United States Army commissioned Lewis Terman of Stanford University to design a similar test for new recruits. Two years later, Terman issued a revised version of Binet's test. Known as the Stanford-Binet Intelligence Scale, it is an IQ test still used today.

Binet concluded that intelligence was a general ability to reason and learn. Others questioned whether intelligence was a general ability or a series of many unrelated aptitudes. English psychologist Charles Spearman believed that in addition to general intelligence, which he called g, there were special aptitudes he labeled s. Competence in a particular area, such as mathematics, would be the product of both general intelligence and the strength of the special aptitude.

Multiple choices, multiple voices: Aptitude tests rally defenders and rouse detractors. Advocates say they stress vital modern-day skills. Critics argue they display cultural bias and cannot gauge creativity.

Attacking the idea of general intelligence in the 1930s, American psychologist Louis Thurstone divided intelligence into seven primary mental abilities (PMAs): memory, numerical ability, reasoning, word fluency, verbal comprehension, perceptual speed and spatial visualization. Two decades later, another broadside was leveled against general intelligence by R. B. Cattell, a British researcher who defined two forms of intelligence. The first, fluid intelligence, was the innate ability to mentally perceive relationships and solve problems. The second, crystallized intelligence, was the collection of mental skills and abilities acquired through experiences. In the 1960s, American psychologist J. P. Guilford proposed his structure-of-intellect model, fragmenting intelligence into 120 separate abilities.

The Spectrum of Intellect

The attempt to define intelligence as a single, general ability has been further complicated by the discovery that the brain's two hemispheres apparently process information differently. Left hemisphere thinking appears to be analytical (taking ideas apart), linear (one step after another) and verbal, while right hemisphere thinking is synthetic (putting ideas together), holistic (grasping relationships in a single step) and imagistic (visual thinking with the "mind's eye"). Although no one employs one hemisphere's mode of thought to the exclusion of the other, writer Aldous Huxley once confessed, "I am and, for as long as I can remember . . . have always been a poor visualizer. Words, even the pregnant words of poets, do not evoke pictures in my mind."

Researchers today question whether we can continue to regard the left hemisphere's gifts of language, science and most mathematics as expressions of intelligence, while placing the abilities of the right hemisphere in the realm of the arts. Says Roger Sperry of the California Institute of Technology: "Right and left hemisphere faculties . . . could make for quite a spectrum of human intellect — from the mechanical or artistic geniuses on the one hand who can hardly express themselves in writing or speech, to the highly articulate individuals at the other extreme who think almost entirely in verbal terms."

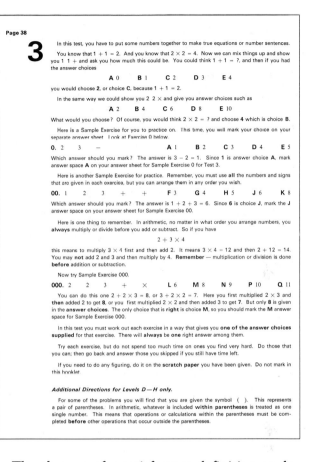

The absence of a satisfactory definition or description of intelligence has often raised the question: What, then, do intelligence tests test? In general, current tests of intelligence measure the verbal, numerical and reasoning skills required by schools and a technological society. Heavily loaded with tasks and questions geared to the brain's left hemisphere, the Stanford-Binet Intelligence Scale, Scholastic Aptitude Test (SAT) and Weschler Adult Intelligence Scale (WAIS) measure our aptitude for convergent thinking, or the ability to logically deduce correct answers. Measured less well, or not at all, by intelligence tests is divergent thinking, the ability to discover new answers, a way of thinking psychologists believe to be crucial to creativity.

Other intellectual abilities not measured by intelligence tests include social intelligence, or the ability to get along with people, musical and artistic aptitudes and the mental gymnastics need-

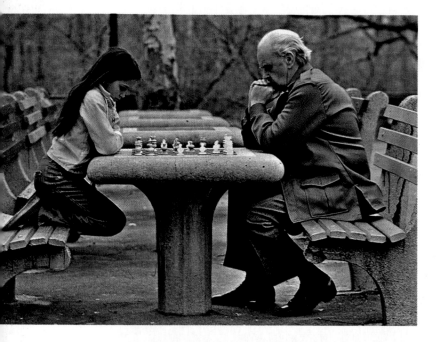

ed to play chess. Intangible human qualities like leadership, motivation and intuition also resist measurement by current tests.

While psychologists and educators have found intelligence tests to be statistically reliable indicators of success in school, these tests have been less useful in predicting success in later life. Concluded Lewis Terman, one of the founding fathers of American IQ testing: "Some aspects of intelligence are so elusive that no tests man has been able to devise have so far enabled us to map them or quantify them."

Testing theoreticians are currently investigating more comprehensive ways of measuring intelligence. One method of inquiry tests reaction time, the time it takes a person to respond to a flashing light or ringing bell. Measured in milliseconds, these responses indirectly gauge how quickly brain cells fire, relax and fire again. Advocates of reaction-time tests believe the quicker the firing patterns, the quicker the mind.

With the aid of computers and the electroencephalograph (EEG), researchers have discovered that sight and sound cause distinctive patterns of electrical activity in the brain. These "fingerprints of the brain" have been compared to IQ data and suggest a relationship between brain-wave patterns and intelligence. Measurements of the brain's electrical activity may one day be useful in testing the intelligence of children too young to take written tests.

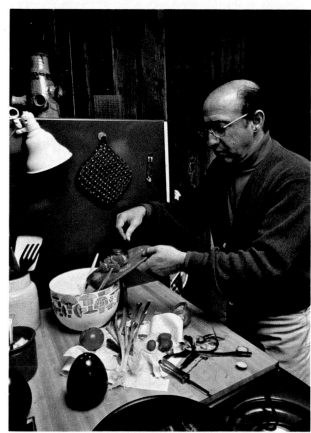

Harvard's David McClelland has taken a different approach to measuring intelligence, one stressing challenges likely to be encountered in life. In an airline-scheduling test he and an associate devised, the test taker has a limited amount of time and money to get from one city to another. The problem has several solutions, but one is more efficient than the others.

Implicit in all the testing and statistical analysis is the assumption that individual intellectual capabilities differ, a fact as undeniable as the existence of the genius and the retardate. More controversial, however, is whether these differences are caused by heredity or environment. In other words, what matters more, the brain one is born with or the world into which that brain is born? Many psychologists believe that heredity

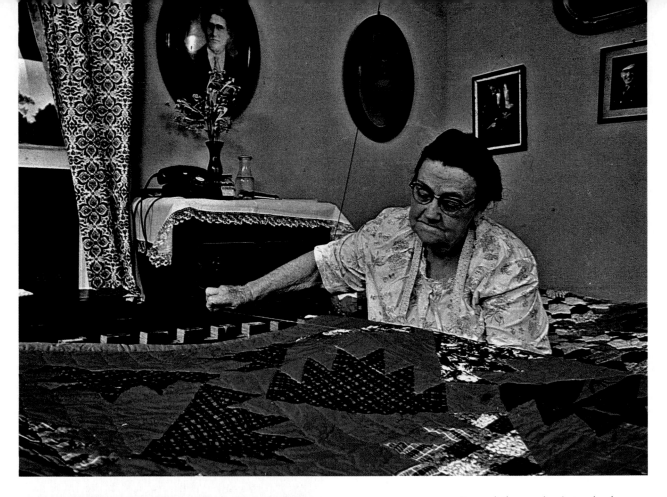

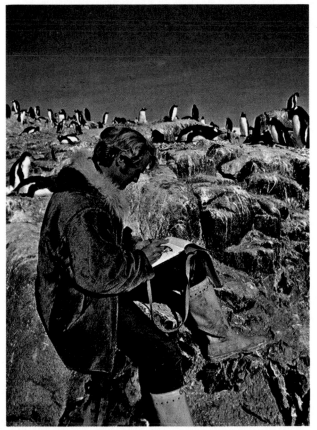

Beyond the reach of standard aptitude tests extends a galaxy of mental feats. Sprung from intuition, channeled by reason, such creative tasks flow from a melding of the mind's many powers. How well a person performs them depends upon an array of factors combining an individual's heredity and environment.

establishes the range of a person's potential intellectual development, while the environment determines the extent of the intellectual development within that range. Although both heredity and environment are essential, it is currently impossible to determine how much each contributes to an individual's intelligence.

The hereditary contribution has been established by studies of identical and fraternal twins. Identical twins have the same genes and, in general, have greater similarities in IQ scores than fraternal twins, whose genetic relationship is more distant. In most cases, the closer the genetic relationship, the closer the tested intelligence.

The environmental contributions to intelligence — nutrition, loving care and attention and intellectual stimulation — have been harder to prove scientifically. The controversy over the relative contributions of heredity and environment has grown bitter over the meaning of a testing statistic: black Americans score, on average, ten to fifteen points lower on IQ tests than whites. In a study released in 1969, psychologist Arthur Jensen suggested that blacks were innately intellectually inferior to whites. Citing the similarity of IQ scores of identical twins raised apart, he argued that hereditary influences far outweighed the socioeconomic factors blamed for the black deficiency — inferior education, poor nutrition, scant prenatal care and IQ tests culturally biased in favor of middle-class whites.

Critics charged that Jensen's research was open to different interpretations, suggesting that intelligence could be enhanced by an enriched environment, enough to erase the fifteen-point deficiency with ease. Further research matching the IQs of black and white children raised together in an upper-middle-class environment indicated no significant intellectual differences between the races. And, as the 1970s drew to a close, one of Jensen's major sources, British psychologist Cyril Burt, was accused by his official biographer of inventing figures and the names of researchers who had supposedly compiled them.

Although the controversy over the relative contributions of heredity and environment endures, many researchers agree with Canadian psychologist Donald Hebb's observation that asking which contributes more to intelligence, heredity or environment, is like asking which contributes more to the area of a field — its length or its width? "Neither," Hebb concluded, "can contribute anything by itself."

From Banal to Sublime

The traditional means of defining and testing intelligence usually exclude perhaps man's most precious mental ability, creativity. Expressions of creativity are more easily agreed upon than its definition. Described by writer Arthur Koestler as "the defeat of habit by originality," creativity requires more than novel insight. The insight must also be fitting. A symphony or a painting must have aesthetic value, and a scientific discovery must be confirmed by experiments.

Requiring intuition and logic, fantasy and craftsmanship, inspiration and perspiration, creative insights are the product of many seemingly opposite ways of thinking. Although scientific discoveries are often thought to be the result of rational, analytical thinking, it appears that the physicist, chemist and mathematician must be no less intuitive than the poet, composer or painter. In a moment of introspection, Albert Einstein observed, "When I examine myself and my methods of thought I come to the conclusion that the gift of fantasy has meant more to me than my talent for absorbing positive knowledge."

On the other hand, artists need more than just inspiration and fantasy to be creative. They must also be rational, self-critical masters of their discipline. Composer Franz Schubert believed the source of Beethoven's genius was his "superb coolness under the fire of creative fantasy." Indeed, Beethoven's sketchbooks show how he laboriously revised his compositions, transforming the banal into the sublime.

One theory divides creativity into four stages. The first stage is preparation. The artist or scientist immerses himself in the problem. The preparation stage requires much of the hard work that usually precedes any creative insight — Einstein spent nearly ten years formulating his special theory of relativity. During the second, an incubation stage of the creative process, the problem is put aside. Ideas, associations and relationships

Jean Piaget

Pioneer of Intellect

In 1920, the Paris laboratories of Alfred Binet sent out a new researcher to see how many five-year-olds could pass a new test of reasoning. The young man, twenty-four-year-old Jean Piaget, was fascinated by those who failed. Why had they?

He discovered a regularity in the children's errors, which seemed systematic. Children of the same age often made the same mistakes, suggesting a similarity in underlying mental structures. He decided to investigate his idea. This detour lasted sixty years — the rest of Piaget's life.

The psychologist talked to children and watched them play. He thought standardized tests were too rigid for studying intelligence, and favored his own judgment to statistics.

Piaget found that children reasoned in a different manner than adults. They had, in his words, "quite different world views, literally different philosophies." He saw the child as an artist who painted a picture of reality based on exploratory collisions with the environment.

The children Piaget studied often were not logical thinkers, but he did not believe them illogical either. A child's reasoning was a different, "pre-logical" view of the world.

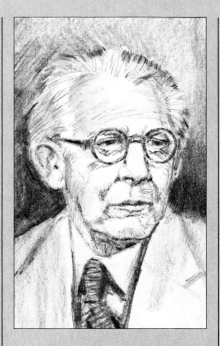

Piaget discovered classes of basic problems children could solve only by growing older. He grouped mental abilities into four chronological stages of development, each built upon the previous one.

During the first stage, from birth until about two years of age, a child explores his environment and gradually becomes aware of his effect on it. Until the approximate age of ten months, a child typically thinks that objects and people he cannot see no longer exist.

In the second stage, lasting from about age two to seven, children begin to think symbolically and indulge in games of fantasy. A stick becomes a gun, and a doll, a "mommy."

Toward the end of this stage, children can understand that the quantity of something remains the same, regardless of the shape. When the contents of two identical glasses, equally full, are poured into a tall thin glass and a short fat glass, the five-year old thinks the tall glass holds more liquid. But a seven-year old correctly reasons that both glasses contain the same amount.

Logical and abstract thinking develop in the third stage, ages seven to twelve. Children use numbers, sort things by size and weight and categorize objects by class — roses, tulips and violets are all flowers.

In the final stage, from ages twelve to fifteen, youngsters think in abstractions. They distinguish between conjecture and reality and understand irony or double-entendre. Piaget theorized that all children go through these stages in the same order and at the same approximate ages.

The Swiss psychologist probably contributed far more than any other researcher to knowledge of man's intellectual development. A reserved and thoughtful man, Piaget possessed the gift of patience and the ability to understand the world as a child sees it.

To the Greeks, creativity was a gift from the Muses, the nine daughters of Zeus and Mnemosyne. At right, nineteenth-century French artist Henri Rousseau invokes the spirit of the poetic muse in his portrait of Marie Laurencin, painter, mistress and inspiration to poet Guillaume Apollinaire. Below, Japanese painter Kyosai depicts Buddhist deity Aizen Myo-o guiding the hand of fellow artist Hayashi Hosen.

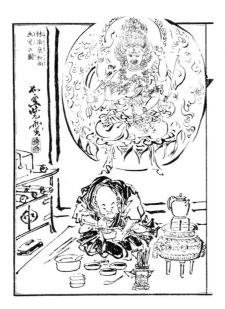

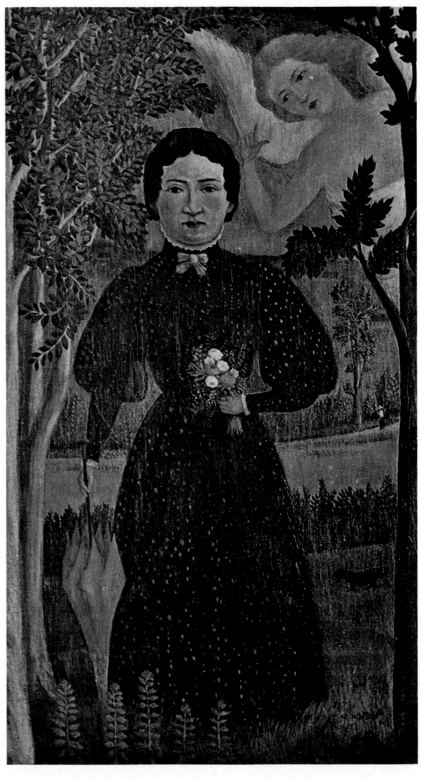

74

percolate beneath the creator's conscious awareness. Many artists and scientists stimulate the incubation period by taking long walks, rides or even by sleeping. The next stage, illumination, is frequently called the "Aha!" response that bursts into the creator's conscious mind, often with startling clarity and impact. One of French mathematician Henri Poincaré's sudden insights occurred while he was boarding a bus: "At the moment when I put my foot on the step the idea came to me, without anything in my former thoughts seeming to have paved the way for it." The fourth and final stage is verification. During this stage, the artist or scientist transcribes his inner vision into the language of his discipline, be it words, equations or musical notes. Because of the clarity and certainty of the insight, many creators regard this step as anticlimactic. Of his music Mozart wrote, "the committing to paper is done quickly enough, for everything is . . . already finished; and it rarely differs on paper from what it was in my imagination."

The creative act, however, does not always happen in such a neat sequence of steps. For poets, writers and composers, the "Aha!" response may be the germinal idea that initiates creative thought. Moreover, many researchers believe creative insights are the result of many overlapping incubations and illuminations that occur as the creative product is refined and developed.

Regardless of the sequence of stages, the preparation and verification stages of creativity tap the logical, verbal strengths of the brain's left hemisphere. The incubation and illumination stages — the heart of the creative process — use the gifts of the brain's intuitive right hemisphere. Composer Aaron Copland's description of his creative process suggests the division of labor between the brain's two hemispheres: "One-half of the personality emotes and dictates while the other half listens and notates. The half that listens had better look the other way, had better simulate a half attention only, for the half that dictates is easily disgruntled and avenges itself for too close inspection by fading entirely away."

The right hemisphere's ability to think in visual and auditory images appears to be crucial to creativity. Free of the shackles of language and

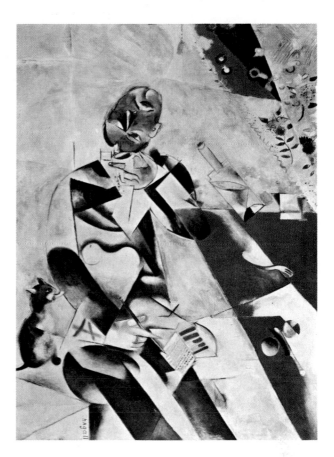

verbal thought, the mute right hemisphere scans, manipulates and develops these images. Wrote Beethoven, "In my head, I begin to elaborate the work in its breadth, its narrowness, its height, its depth and, since I am aware of what I want to do, the underlying idea never deserts me. It rises, it grows, I hear and see the image in front of me from every angle, as if it had been cast."

The right hemisphere's capacity for visual imagery is apparently no less important for scientific creativity. In a letter to mathematician Jacques Hadamard, Einstein wrote that "the words or the language, as they are written or spoken, do not seem to play any role in my mechanism of thought. The psychical entities which seem to serve as elements of thought are certain signs and more or less clear images which can be 'voluntarily' reproduced and combined . . . . this combinatory play seems to be the essential feature in productive thought."

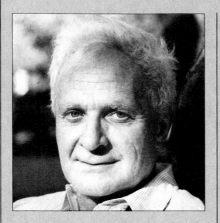

Stephen Spender
English poet:

"Inspiration is the beginning of a poem and it is also its final goal. It is the first idea which drops into the poet's mind and it is the final idea which he at last achieves in words. In between this start and this winning post there is the hard race, the sweat and toil. . . . One line is given to the poet by God or by nature, the rest he has to discover for himself."

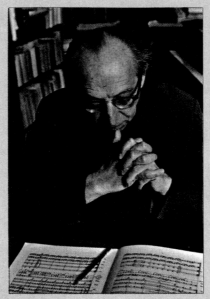

Aaron Copland
American composer:

"The source of the germinal idea is the one phase in creation that resists rational explanation. All we know is that the moment of possession is the moment of inspiration. . . . Whence it comes, or in what manner it comes or how long its duration one can never foretell. Inspiration may be a form of superconsciousness, or perhaps of subconsciousness — I wouldn't know; but I am sure that it is the antithesis of self-consciousness."

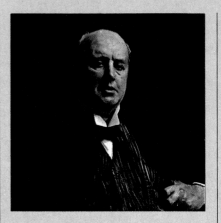

Henry James
American novelist:

"Most of the stories straining to shape under my hand have sprung from a single small seed, a seed as minute and windblown as that casual hint for *The Spoils of Poynton* dropped unwitting by my neighbour, a mere floating particle in the stream of talk. . . . Such is the interesting truth about the stray suggestion, the wandering word, the vague echo, at touch of which the novelist's imagination winces as at the prick of some sharp point: its virtue is all in its needlelike quality, the power to penetrate as finely as possible."

patience and discipline collapses; ideas languish and die. Often coming at serendipitous moments — during a walk, a dream, a desperate gazing upon blank canvas — inspiration salves wounds of *self-doubt opened by hours of seemingly fruitless thought. A goal that gives the journey meaning, it affirms the mind's pursuit — and in so doing awes those that know its power best:*

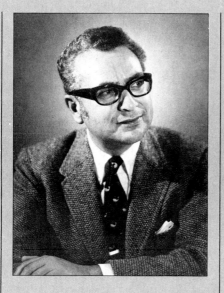

Murray Gell-Mann
American physicist:

"One of my ideas came in a slip of the tongue. I was getting up at a seminar — one person had just put forward a theory, and I was explaining why his theory was wrong, why it didn't work — and while I was explaining it, I happened to blurt out the correct way to do it. Just a slip of the tongue. And I recognized immediately that that would solve the problem."

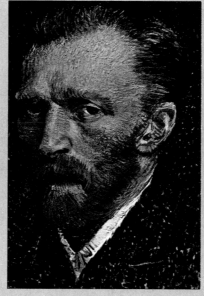

Vincent van Gogh
Dutch artist:

"How I paint . . . *I do not know myself*. I sit down with a white board before the spot that strikes me, I look at what is before me, I say to myself that that white board must become something; I come back dissatisfied; I put it away, and when I have rested a little, I go to look at it with a kind of fear. Then I am still dissatisfied, because I have still too clearly in my mind that splendid scene of nature. . . . I see that nature has told me something, has spoken to me, and that I have put it down in shorthand. . . . Now I feel myself on the high seas; the painting must be continued with all the strength I can give to it."

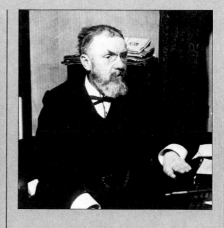

Jules Henri Poincaré
French mathematician:

"For fifteen days I strove to prove that there could not be any functions like those I have since called Fuchsian functions. I was then very ignorant; every day I seated myself at my work table, stayed an hour or two, tried a great number of combinations and reached no results. One evening, contrary to my custom, I drank black coffee and could not sleep. Ideas rose in crowds; I felt them collide until pairs interlocked, so to speak, making a stable combination. By the next morning I had established the existence of a class of Fuchsian functions. . . . I had only to write out the results, which took but a few hours."

*Creativity springs from intuition
and logic. An African headdress,
Picasso's* Woman on a Sofa *and
Roy Lichtenstein's* Woman With
Flowered Hat *are expressions of
creativity through a common theme.*

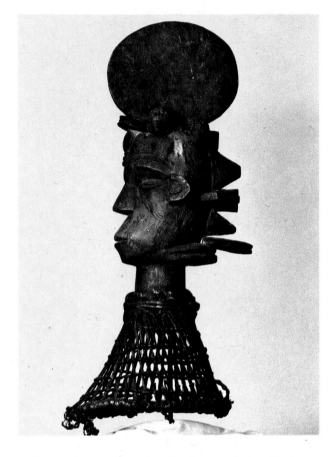
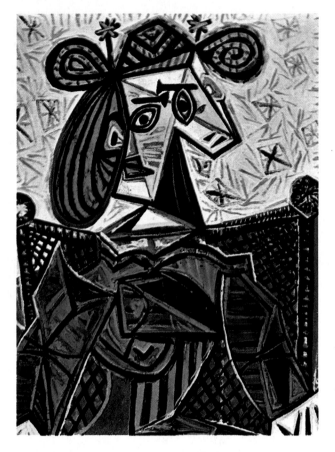

Beyond a certain level of tested intelligence, there seems to be little relationship between IQ and creativity. Tests designed to measure imagination reveal that the highly creative are less "stimulus bound" than others who may have a higher IQ. When shown a picture and asked to explain it, creative people usually exercise their powers of fantasy. Those less imaginative adhere more rigidly to the picture's visual content.

Creative people are as seemingly contradictory as the creative act. At once self-centered and self-critical, the highly creative often see the strange in the ordinary and the ordinary in the strange. Picasso made a bull from the seat and handlebars of a bicycle, and Mozart composed elaborate variations on the children's tune "Twinkle, Twinkle Little Star." The highly creative are intensely observant; artists are good witnesses at the scene of an accident. Creative people thrive on complexity and confusion. To researcher Frank Barron, they are both "crazier and saner than the average person," a sentiment echoed in a verse penned by Albert Einstein:

A thought that sometimes makes me hazy:
Am I or are the others crazy?

The association of creativity with mental instability is at least as old as classical Greek thought. Socrates believed that "No one without a touch of the muse's madness will enter into the temple of art." And Sigmund Freud, the father of psychoanalysis, believed that unresolved conflicts were the source of creative activity. But today, many researchers regard creativity as a sign of mental health. The creative person's flexibility, independence, perseverance and tolerance for ambiguity are characteristics of a well-adjusted individual. Too, the integration of left and right hemisphere thinking in creative activity often produces a sense of psychological wholeness.

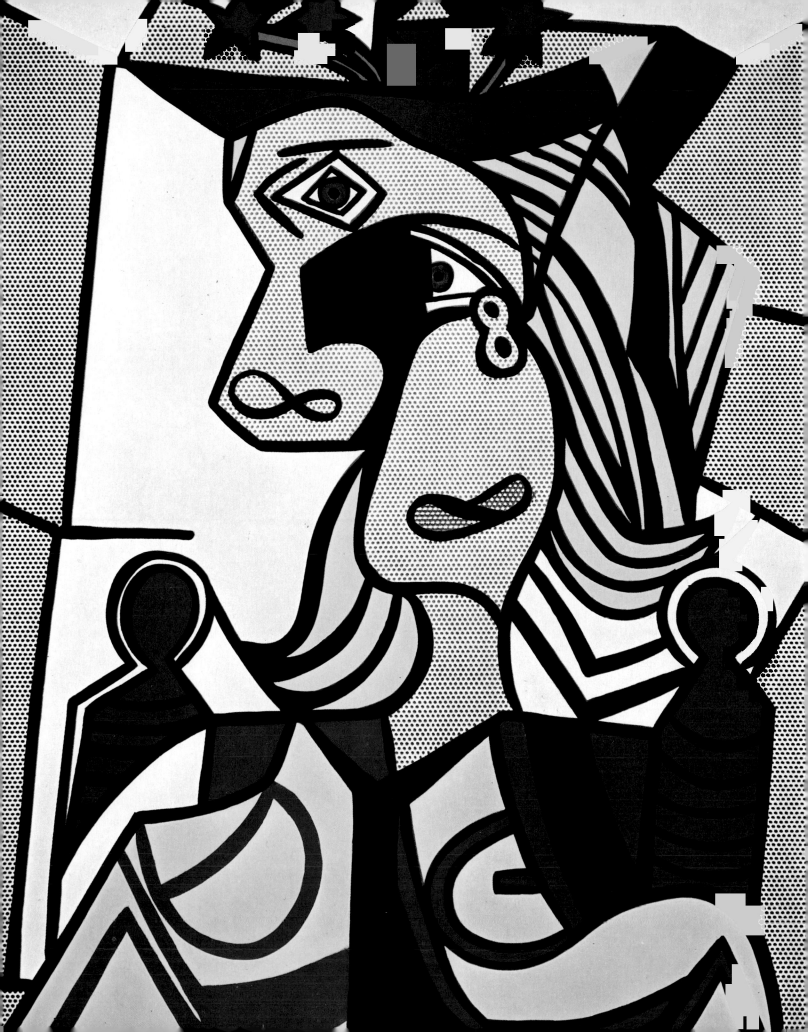

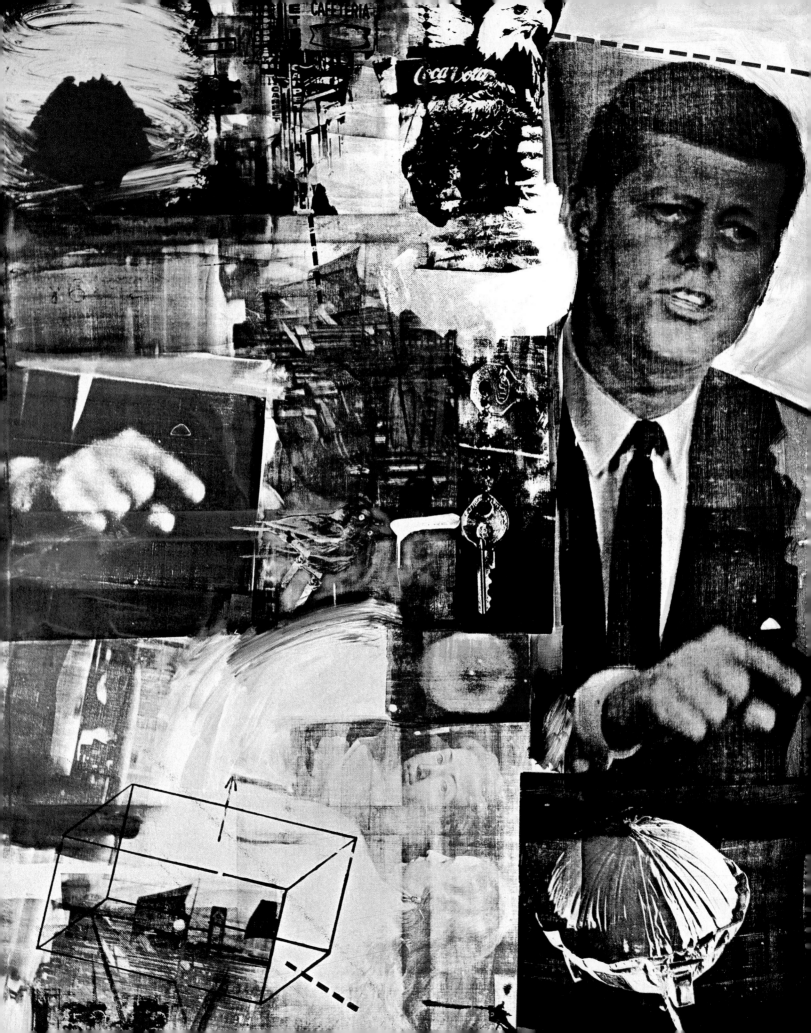

Chapter 6

Remembrance of Things Past

In seeking to understand the mind of man, philosopher John Locke compared it to "white paper, void of all characters, without any ideas." How then, he wondered, "comes it to be furnished? Whence comes it by that vast store, which the busy and boundless fancy of man has painted on it with an almost endless variety? . . . To this I answer in one word . . . experience." Memory is man's record of experience. The ability to remember is essential to human individuality, tying a person's past to his present and creating a continuing sense of identity.

But as the White Queen said to Alice in Lewis Carroll's *Through the Looking Glass*: "It's a poor sort of memory that works only backwards." By drawing on the past, man also prepares for the future. This power of prediction is "the ultimate goal of the evolution of the nervous system," believes biologist Colin Blakemore.

The systems of mind that overcome the experience of the moment and create a continuing flow of consciousness have intrigued and perplexed man for centuries. As our technology has progressed so have our analogies for the mechanisms of the brain. Human memory has been compared to a library, a computer, even a hologram. But one of the simplest and most enduring metaphors for memory was put forth by Sigmund Freud.

The famous Viennese analyst compared memory to a child's toy, the "Magic Slate," made of wax-coated cardboard, wax paper and clear celluloid. The pressure marks of a stylus show up as dark lines on the surface of the pad. Lifting the layers of celluloid and wax paper from the base erases the dark lines. But the writing has not entirely vanished: the original impressions remain embedded in the waxy surface of the cardboard. "Thus," thought Freud, the toy "provides not only a receptive surface that can be used over and over again, like a slate, but also permanent traces of what has been written. . . . It solves the

Memory weaves through Robert Rauschenberg's oil, Buffalo. *Adept at storing the trivial and the staggering, memory is the force that gives unity to man's life. The vault of all knowledge, it enables man to organize and learn from his experience. Memory forms a brilliant collage of the past, adds perspective to the present and colors the future.*

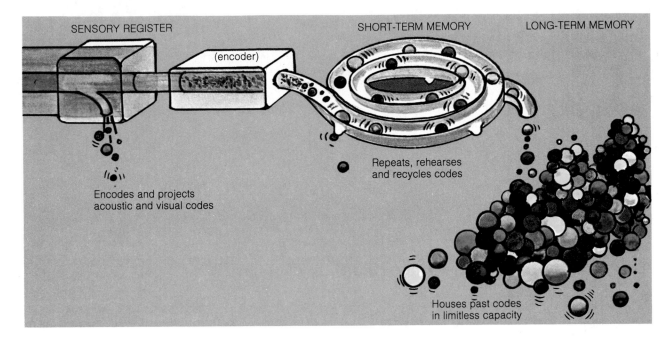

SENSORY REGISTER (encoder) SHORT-TERM MEMORY LONG-TERM MEMORY

Encodes and projects acoustic and visual codes

Repeats, rehearses and recycles codes

Houses past codes in limitless capacity

problem of combining the two functions by dividing them between two separate but interrelated component parts or systems." In human memory, these two interrelated systems are known as short-term and long-term memory.

Before an event can be stored in the memory, it must be experienced in some way by the brain. As information flows in from the senses, the brain briefly retains the entire stimulus. The image of a painting fleetingly haunts the retina when the eye is closed; a musical note echoes in the brain as the flute player pauses for breath. This mechanism, called the sensory register, holds an image for less than a second and retains a sound for no more than four seconds — long enough for the brain's perceptual systems to act on them. The register records a vast amount of potential information, but only a small amount filters into the short-term memory. The boundaries of human attention limit the information a person can handle; some images, though they peripherally register on the senses, vanish from awareness like breath on a windowpane.

Short-term memory retains information long enough for the mind to grasp it. Unless an individual makes an effort to remember an item, it remains in the short-term memory for less than a

minute. Most of the information is recorded in verbal form. The letter *s*, for example, is retained as the sound "ess" instead of the shape S. If an item cannot be retained in a verbal form, it is generally held as a visual image. Short-term memory holds a limited amount of information. It stores an average of seven items (the length of a telephone number) at a time, and erases older items as new ones are added.

If an individual wants to retain an item in the short-term memory for more than a moment, he must rehearse it. A man wanting to reserve a table at a restaurant looks up the telephone number and repeats it to himself before he makes the call. By focusing his attention on the number, the man limits other information entering his short-term memory and prevents the number from being erased. If he dials it frequently, he may find after a while that he simply remembers it. The number has been transferred to a more accessible reference — long-term memory.

Man's permanent memory houses an astounding range of information — from images of childhood to the rules of language. In short, it stores all of man's knowledge about himself and his world. In order to retain so much information, long-term memory employs a more sophisticated

Karl Lashley
In Search of the Engram
Wilder Penfield
Unlocking the Secrets of Memory

Like pirates seeking treasure, scientists have long sought an answer to the question posed, among other places, in the Bible's Book of Job:

For there is a mine for silver,
And a place for gold which
they refine. . . .
But wisdom, where shall it be
found?
And where is the place of understanding?

Beginning in 1917, neuropsychologist Karl Lashley conducted a hunt for this elusive treasure. He aimed to find the brain's engram — the elusive, permanent traces of memory.

Lashley trained animals, usually rats, to perform a variety of tasks, then systematically removed portions of their brains. He found that he could damage the animals' visual and motor abilities but never completely destroy their memory of tasks testing vision and movement, even when he removed large portions of the cortex.

Publishing "In Search of the Engram" in 1950, Lashley said his studies "yielded a good bit of information about what and where the memory trace is not." He had "discovered nothing directly of the real nature of the engram." Memory, he theorized, was not located in any one region of the

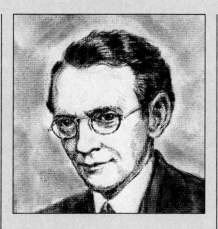

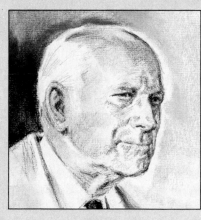

brain nor linked throughout by any specific physical structure. It must therefore be equipotential — located with equal power at all points in the brain. Lashley concluded, "There is no great excess of cells which can be reserved as the seat of special memories."

At almost the same time that Lashley's research was indicating there was no memory engram, another investigator, Canadian neurosurgeon Wilder Penfield, was producing evidence to the contrary.

Penfield began electrically stimulating the exposed brains of epileptic patients in the late 1920s to determine the location of abnormal brain tissue and the functions its removal might endanger.

When Penfield probed a region of the temporal lobes, lying on each side of the brain, the patients' responses took him by surprise.

One patient heard a voice singing and remembered the name of the song, "Oh Marie, Oh Marie." Another saw himself talking with his friends in South Africa. Hearing an orchestra playing, a woman hummed the music for Penfield. A boy heard his mother talking on the telephone and, after several touches of the probe, could repeat her entire conversation.

All in all, forty epileptic patients recalled similar memories. The temporal region, he theorized, must be "part of an automatic mechanism which scans the record of the past," linking the cortex to deeper brain structures thought to be involved in memory. "In the vast circuitry of the human brain," Penfield confidently wrote, "the evidence of an engram . . . is clear."

method of storage than short-term memory. As psychologist Ernest Kent describes it, "Short-term memory allows us to recall what was said verbatim, while recall from long-term memory generally involves paraphrase." This suggests that we store permanent memories in terms of their meaning, retaining concepts and relationships instead of words themselves.

Are they two independent systems of memory or are they somehow interconnected? The most popular theory, advanced by Canadian psychologist Donald Hebb in 1949, proposes a connection between the two types of memory. In Hebb's view, short-term memory is an active, or dynamic, memory: sight or sound sets off a reverberating pattern of nerve impulses in the brain. The impulses circle a closed loop of connected neurons, freezing an instant of time long enough for the brain to perceive it. But the neurons fire for only a short time, so dynamic memory will fade away unless a more permanent, structural trace is made. This structural trace, or engram, would correspond to long-term memory.

The Indelible Engram
Psychologist Charles Furst compares Hebb's two processes of memory storage to the flow of water down a hill: "Dynamic traces would be like rivulets of water. . . . When the water stops, the pattern of rivulets disappears. But if the water runs long enough, then the rivulets cut channels and wear the pattern into the hillside, so that a permanent 'memory' of it has been formed." Short-term memories could thus be converted into long-term memories. If the nerve impulses circle their selected pathways long enough, they could leave behind an indelible memory trace.

The structure of this trace, or engram, remains a matter of speculation. Many theories have been advanced, including the one that memory is coded in proteins or smaller chains of molecules. In the 1960s, the University of Michigan's James McConnell trained planaria, small flatworms, to turn away from light. He cut up the trained worms and fed them to untrained worms. This group learned their task more quickly than another group fed untrained worms. McConnell reasoned that memory must therefore be stored

chemically. In pursuing the chemical basis of memory, researchers discovered that a laboratory animal's neurons contained more RNA, or ribonucleic acid, after learning took place. RNA, present in all cells, relays genetic information and builds proteins. Preventing or reducing the production of RNA impaired a test animal's ability to learn. But when the production of RNA was enhanced through chemical injection, the animal showed an improvement in learning.

Scientists soon realized, however, that RNA itself was not the key to memory. In the 1970s, Georges Ungar of the Baylor College of Medicine in Houston conducted experiments exploring the possibility that proteins made by RNA affect specific types of memory and mental functions. Although rats are normally nocturnal, Ungar trained them to avoid entering a darkened corner of a specially designed box. He analyzed extracts from their brains and found a new protein he named scotophobin, meaning "fear of darkness." In testing the protein's effects, Ungar found that only part of it — a smaller chain of molecules called a peptide — seemed to affect learning. He injected other rats with a synthetic form created from the peptide's basic elements. The synthetic scotophobin had the same effect. Ungar's findings suggested that a specific chemical might be linked to every learned skill. Other researchers produced similar results in goldfish, thus indicating a universal coding of the substance.

A Memory Network
But the most influential theory, again by Hebb, proposes that memories are fixed in the nerve pathways themselves. Hebb suggested that the continuous flow of nerve impulses along a pathway or loop alters the synaptic connections in some way, perhaps causing new synapses to grow or altering those that already exist. When the electrical activity dies down, the new connections remain, creating a nerve network that stores a specific memory. Activating one or two neurons in the chain will tend to trigger the others and thereby bring the memory back to mind. Hebb's theory holds that it takes a certain amount of time for long-term memories to become fixed in the brain. During this period, a

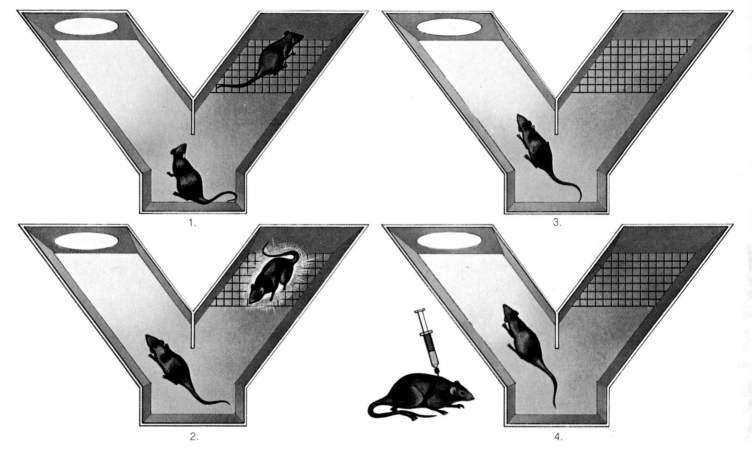

1.

2.

3.

4.

memory exists as short-term electrical activity, capable of being disrupted and lost forever.

The imprinting of permanent memory, it seems, is linked to a specific part of the brain. In 1953, a young man called H. M. underwent an operation for epilepsy. The surgeon removed the hippocampus, a part of his brain thought to be causing the seizures. Although cured of epilepsy, H. M. could no longer store permanent memories. Old memories remained intact. His short-term memory also continued to function. But he would read the same magazine time after time, with no memory of ever having done so. New acquaintances were forever strangers; he could not remember them from one meeting to the next. He was a prisoner of the moment. "Every day is alone in itself," he noted, "whatever enjoyment I've had, and whatever sorrow I've had."

If man had to scan the full contents of his memory for information, the question "What is

Released into a box with dark and light areas, the nocturnal rat naturally seeks a darkened corner (1). But electric shock conditions it to avoid this corner (2) and causes the production of a new peptide linked to the experience (3). An untrained rat, injected with a synthetic form of the peptide, also develops aversion to darkness (4). From such experiments, memory was thought to be stored in brain chemicals.

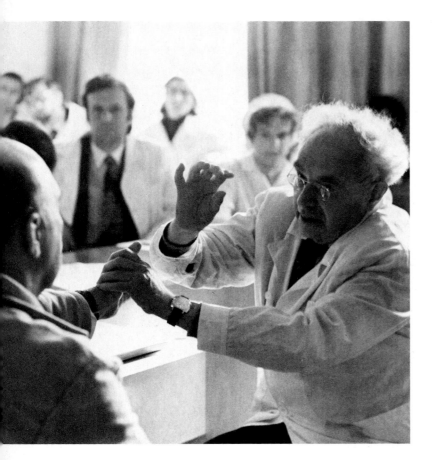

A. R. Luria, Soviet psychologist, gained world renown from studies of patients with severe brain injuries that had stripped them of memory. Luria helped them as they struggled to piece together their shattered world, and added to the knowledge of brain localization. His patients deeply touched him. They fought for life, he wrote, "with a skill psychologists cannot help envying."

your name?" might take hundreds of years to answer. Like a library, the brain has a method of cross-referencing its material. It tags memories with direct associations called retrieval cues that work like indexes to help find information. A walk along the seashore can stir up memories of a vacation spent at the beach; so can a picture of the ocean, the sight of a gull or a poem about the sea. People returning to their childhood home after many years often report feeling "flooded with memories." Scent also evokes powerful memories. A whiff of familiar perfume can stir up not only thoughts of an acquaintance, but feelings as well. Every place, every moment, is a link to the past. Memory provides the transport.

Most retrieval cues work unconsciously, following the many thoughts the mind pursues throughout the day. But retrieval cues are also used deliberately. A person asked to remember his activities on a specific day might look at a calendar to jog his memory, or mentally reconstruct the events hour by hour. Soon, his memory of the day takes shape, like a dream apparition rising into consciousness. While the importance of remembering is obvious, the value of forgetting might not seem so apparent. "If we remembered everything, we should . . . be as ill as if we remembered nothing," speculated imaginative nineteenth-century philosopher William James.

The Man Who Could Not Forget

Some thirty years later, in the 1920s, a Russian newspaperman — known to science as S. — proved the horror of James's conjecture. S.'s memory astonished the Soviet psychologist A. R. Luria. After a series of tests, Luria concluded, "I simply had to admit that the capacity of his memory *had no distinct limits*; that I had been unable to perform what one would think was the simplest task a psychologist can do: measure the capacity of an individual's memory." S. effortlessly recalled long tables of numbers or words, each with as many as seventy items. Many years later when Luria retested him, S. recalled these same tables — in the original order, backwards and diagonally. Plagued by his memory, S. had to devise tricks to forget. He would conjure up a mental canvas and then hang it over images he no longer wanted to remember. To rid himself of a list of numbers, he would write them on an imaginary blackboard and then erase them.

Unlike most people, who remember in both words and images, S. remembered in images alone. Requiring three or four seconds to "imprint" each image in his memory, he then read them with his "mind's eye." He could make these images bigger or smaller, alter their perspective and move them around. He would imagine walking a familiar Moscow street. As he walked, he would distribute the items around landmarks. He might place a pencil near a fence, a banner on a building, a shoe in a window. This technique was not foolproof, however. He once omitted the word *egg* from a list of memorized items because he had mentally placed it next to a white wall. When he called up the image of the street, he failed to notice the egg because it blended in with the wall. S. solved the problem by moving the egg to a contrasting backdrop and adding a mental street light.

More remarkable, S.'s memory was synesthetic. A rare phenomenon, synesthesia caused him to involuntarily experience mixed sensations of sight, sound, touch, taste and smell. Faithfully recording what he sensed of the world, S. remembered "cold sounds" and "rough colors." Once, when Luria asked him if he could find his way back to the research institute, S. nonchalantly replied, "Come, now. How could I possibly forget? After all, here's this fence. It has such a salty taste . . . such a sharp, piercing sound."

To those who did not know him well, S. seemed slow-witted. Simple conversations often confused him. Every word ignited an explosion of multisensory images that sent his mind off on tangents. He could not easily grasp such abstract ideas as infinity. And despite his prodigious memory, S. had a limited capacity for logical thought. He changed jobs frequently, eventually performing his bizarre power for audiences.

Aside from such rare cases, forgetting is commonplace. Without this ability, man's mind would be as cluttered with useless trivia as S.'s was. One psychologist who studied her own memory for six years concluded that while memory does regularly lose bits of information, it

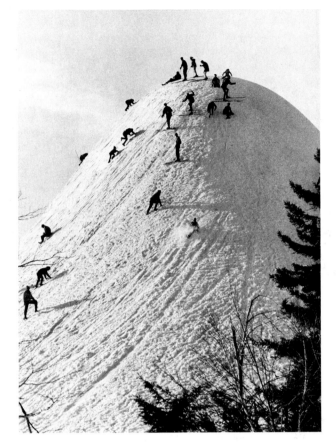

Researchers use the above photograph to test eidetic imagery, the ability to mentally recreate a complete visual experience. Commonly called photographic memory, it occurs mostly in young children but becomes relatively rare after puberty. After studying this picture for thirty seconds, some subjects can recall the exact number of branches on the evergreen tree.

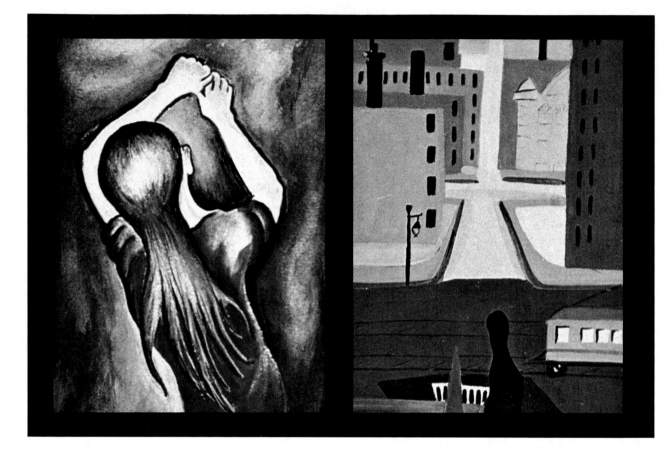

tends to retain important material. Memory, it seems, undergoes a continual spring cleaning.

The interference theory holds that stored memories can compete with each other. Interference may occur when older memories block the storing of new memory, or when new information blocks out older memories. Many people have found that sleep or quiet reflection helps them retain new information, perhaps by preventing interference. Not a new idea, the great Renaissance master Leonardo noted "the praiseworthy exercise" of lying "in bed in the dark to go over again in the imagination the outlines of the forms you have been studying."

The brain cannot retrieve what it has not stored. "The true art of memory," wrote Samuel Johnson, "is the art of attention." Psychologist Eric Klinger of the University of Minnesota has uncovered a revealing characteristic about man's attention. For more than seven years, he studied the attention spans of his students. He asked them to write their thoughts every time a buzzer sounded. Klinger concluded that most people actually daydream about one-third of their waking time. He theorizes that daydreaming might really "be our normal mode of thought" and that "when we direct our thoughts the remaining two-thirds of the time . . . we have to make a special effort to do so."

Even the best memory is imperfect, changing shape and content over time. Memories are individual perceptions. Ten people who witness a crime may remember ten different versions of it. Through the process called constructive error, a person may combine actual recollections with suppositions and inferences to build a more complete yet false memory. Constructive error makes childhood memories grow more brilliant, more detailed with time. As an individual grows older and learns more about a specific event, the new

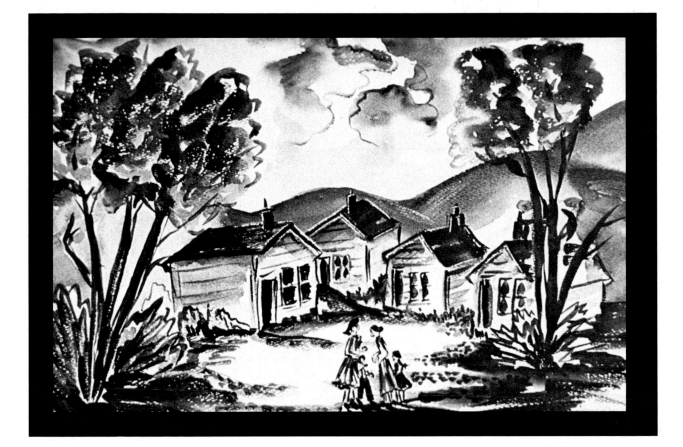

information becomes a part of the original re-membered event. Memory seems to be not only a guardian but a weaver of the past.

Without memory, time would be a meaning-less abstraction and every routine experience a venture into the unknown. One woman known as Sybil possessed sixteen distinct personalities. From childhood on, she would experience long blackouts when the personalities took control of her consciousness. After many years of therapy, her personalities finally merged into one. Only then did she experience the constant flow of time. Her new-found memory continually amazed and delighted her. "Just think, I've been here almost a year now," she wrote to a friend. "It is the first continuous year of my life. It's amazing how days fit neatly into weeks and weeks into months that I can look back on and remember." To patients once deprived of memo-ry, its return gives them a future as well as a past.

Sybil, a woman with sixteen personalities, noted of one that "she has robbed me of my past." In control of her consciousness, many of them shared common interests, stored in memories beyond Sybil's reach. Several were artists whose drawings and paintings aided in her recovery. The depressed Marcia painted the self-portrait at left. A fearful, angry Peggy, in the center painting, portrayed Sybil's mother as a dark, powerful figure, while the home-loving Mary shows Sybil and her mother with childhood friends in the pastoral watercolor above.

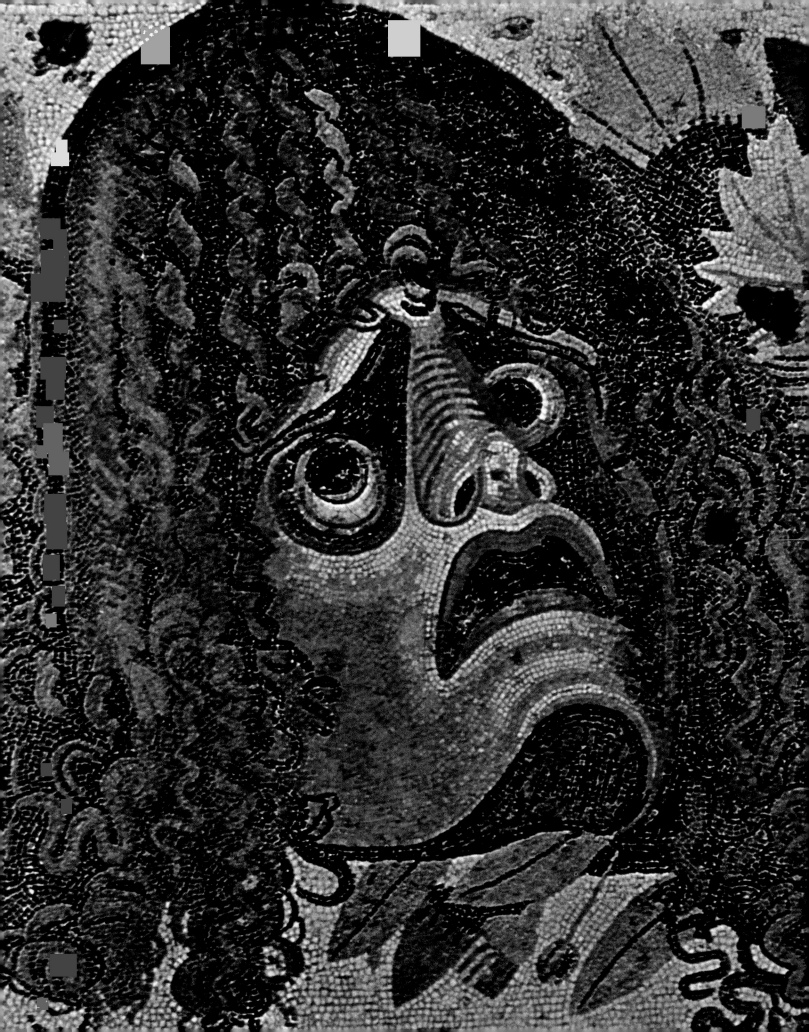

Chapter 7

The Feeling Brain

For centuries, the brain has been regarded primarily as an organ of intellect and cold logic. The pulse of feelings — unruly emotions, sensual cravings and instincts were ascribed to other organs of the body. Sentiment was thought to be the heart's confection. Hunger seemed to emanate from the stomach; sexual desire, from the loins.

In reality, our passions and our drives are as much the brain's creation as are intellect and reason. They are all brought to life in a small amphitheater of tissue known as the limbic system. Inside a collection of parts that make up roughly one-fifth of the brain's area, the cold world of reality is transformed into a bubbling caldron of human feelings. The forces of fear, elation, grief, anger and lust arise from this most primitive region of the brain that evolved long ago.

The limbic system constitutes the middle layer of what neuroscientist Paul MacLean calls the "triune brain." In his model, the brain is composed of three concentric layers, each representing a different stage of evolution. The most primitive layer is the brainstem, sometimes called the reptilian brain because it is found in all vertebrates from reptiles to man. The brainstem regulates the vital body functions of heartbeat and respiration. Surrounding the reptilian brain is the limbic system, or old mammalian brain. The cerebrum, the most recent layer to evolve, swells around the limbic system. In man, the cerebrum is the center for higher thought processes.

The limbic system is also considered primitive because it is found in almost the same form in all mammals. So extensive are its connections to the nerves processing information about smell that scientists once called it the rhinencephalon, meaning "nose brain." But since the keenness of man's sense of smell is not as great as other animals', many scientists wondered why the limbic system occupied so large a part of the brain.

Medusa, terrible monster and goddess of Greek mythology, captures the strength of human emotions in this first-century B.C. mosaic from Pompeii. Impulses surging from the limbic region of the brain imbue our lives with feeling.

91

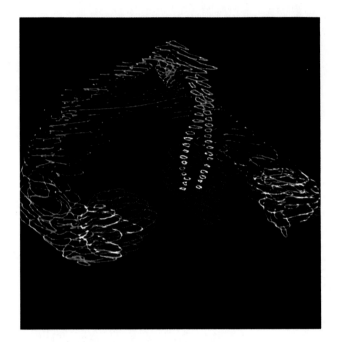

A computer-generated, three-dimensional image of the limbic system recreates its shape. This display from the laboratory of Robert Livingston at the University of California at San Diego was made by computer analysis of tissue-thin cross sections cut on a device called a microtome.

The limbic system, through extensive neural links, works with both the cerebrum above and the brainstem below. Its connections with the brainstem seem to help in maintaining a state of emotional balance and alertness. Connections between the limbic system and the cerebrum permit an interplay between reason and emotion. Generally, the two processes work in harmony, but the balance can be easily upset. The limbic system can become so highly activated that it overwhelms rational thought, making a person speechless with fury or joy. Through conscious control, a person can resist the urge to eat or drink, fight back tears or suppress sexual desire.

Linked together, the various parts of the limbic system encircle the brainstem like a wishbone. The hippocampus, fornix and parahippocampal gyrus make up the swollen lower tip of each fork. Attached to the interior tip of both forks is the almond-shaped amygdala. Suspended over each of the lower forks are two rounded structures — the septum pellucidum and mammillary body. Surrounding this wishbonelike structure, the cingulate gyrus sweeps down in a graceful arc, meeting the parahippocampal gyrus below.

Interwoven throughout the limbic system, nerve pathways send a continuous flow of electrochemical impulses that direct human drives and emotions. The hippocampus, essential in learning, converts information from short-term to long-term memory. It constantly checks information relayed to the brain by the senses and compares it to experience. The thalamus, an egg-shaped mass perched above the brainstem, bonds to limbic structures through abundant nerve links. A major relay station, it analyzes and passes information from sensory and motor nerves to the brain.

Nestled between the thalamus above and the brainstem below, lies a small cluster of nerve cells called the hypothalamus. Only the size of a thumb tip, its blood supply is one of the richest in the entire body. From it arise feelings of pleasure, punishment, hunger, thirst, sexual arousal, aggression and rage. "Had its functions been known in medieval times," muses writer Nigel Calder, "the hypothalamus would no doubt have been designated the Devil's playground."

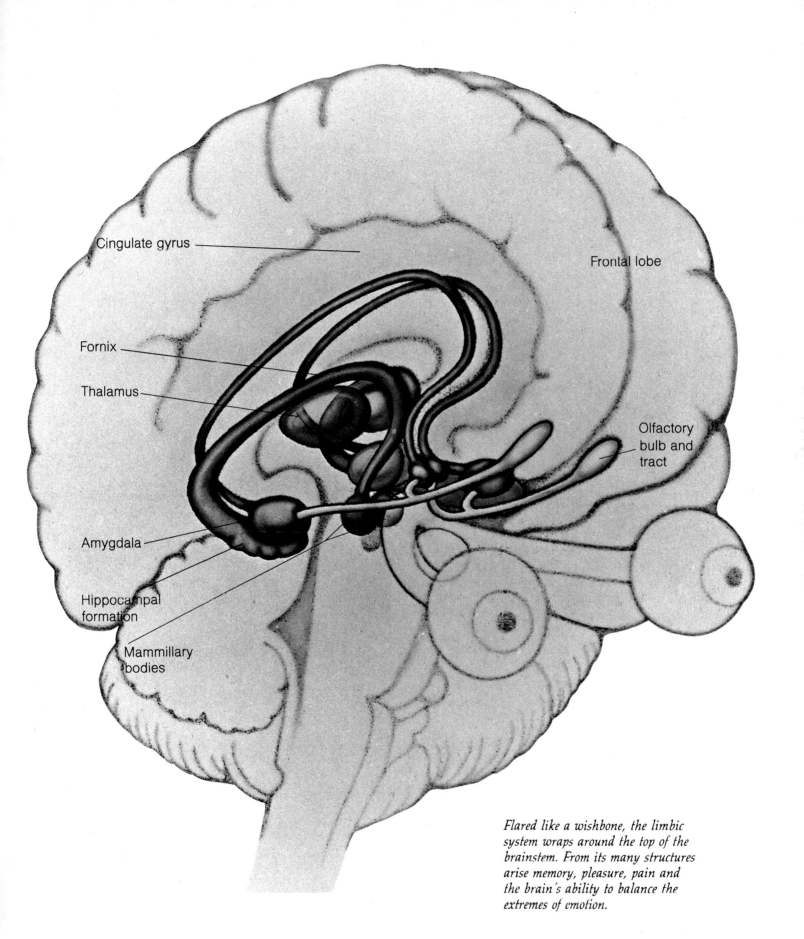

Cingulate gyrus

Frontal lobe

Fornix

Thalamus

Olfactory bulb and tract

Amygdala

Hippocampal formation

Mammillary bodies

Flared like a wishbone, the limbic system wraps around the top of the brainstem. From its many structures arise memory, pleasure, pain and the brain's ability to balance the extremes of emotion.

*Electrode's needle point, left, enables
a brain surgeon to alter behavior
and emotions. Probes set through the
skull, opposite, can stimulate
targeted tissue or destroy pain-
producing areas with strong current.*

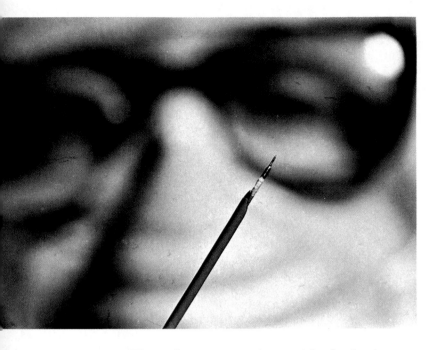

Through its connections with the brainstem, the hypothalamus maintains homeostasis, the body's internal equilibrium. It keeps body temperature at roughly 98.6 degrees by means of a complex thermostat system that reacts to messages from temperature-sensing skin receptors and impulses from heat-sensitive nerve cells near the front of the hypothalamus.

Hunger and thirst centers in the hypothalamus serve as the body's appestat. Here, tiny receptors, sense organs, track glucose levels in the blood. When supplies of this vital energy food plummet, the hypothalamus generates hunger pangs. Hypothalamic disorders may cause compulsive eating or loss of interest in food, depending on the particular hypothalamic region affected. The sensation of thirst arises through receptors measuring the salt level in the blood. With this sophisticated sensing system, the body constantly balances and replenishes itself.

Pathways of Pain and Pleasure

Much of our knowledge of the limbic system stems from electrical stimulation of the brain, or ESB. More than a century ago, German physicians Eduard Hitzig and Gustav Fritsch applied a mild current to electrodes implanted in the cerebral cortex of a dog. Thus they found the brain centers that controlled specific motor functions.

In 1928, neurosurgeon Wilder Penfield began using ESB in operations for epilepsy and other human brain disorders. Probing the cerebrum, he elicited sounds and visions. Others later discovered that stimulation of the limbic system in patients provoked reactions ranging from anger and anxiety to euphoria, sexual interest and states of deep relaxation. "It would thus seem," MacLean wrote, "that the raw stuff of emotion is built into the circuitry" of the limbic system.

Above the hypothalamus is the amygdala, a mass of nerve cells thought to be related to feelings of rage and aggression. Electrical stimulation of the amygdala can incite fury. Its surgical removal turned a once raging, suicidal epileptic into a childlike, docile and apathetic man. But scientists are still not certain of the amygdala's precise role. Its removal does not always produce docility, nor does stimulation uniformly induce rage. Experiments suggest that the amygdala, like the hypothalamus, may possess sites for diverse emotions. One patient with a long history of violence and spells of rage screamed that he was "going wild" when doctors stimulated his amygdala. Yet when the current was applied only three millimeters away, he felt extremely relaxed, describing his mood as one of "detachment." British neurologist Peter Nathan hypothesizes that "the crude display of the rage reaction is organized by the hypothalamus. The amygdala brings subtlety into the reaction, modifying it according to the rapidly changing circumstances resulting from the aggressive behavior."

The septum, linked to the hypothalamus at the front of the limbic ring, appears to contain yet another limbic pleasure center. When ESB experimenter Robert Heath of Tulane University stimulated this limbic region of a man suffering from severe depression, the patient instantly felt cheerful. Cancer victims have received instant pain relief from septal stimulation. Heath has also found that brain-wave activity in the septal area intensifies during sexual arousal. Septal disorders, he believes, might account for anhedonia, an emotional disturbance which renders an individual incapable of experiencing pleasure.

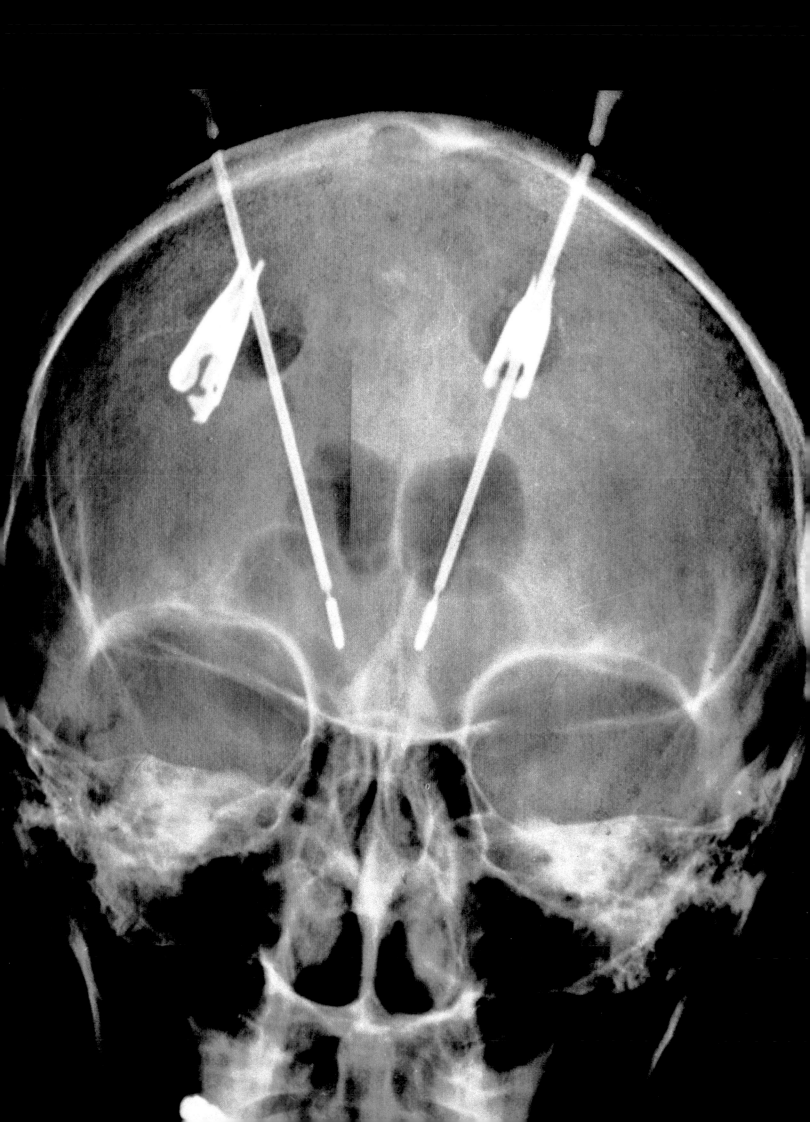

Walter Hess

Electrifying Brain Research

Even at the age of eighty-six, Walter Hess had a fascination for electricity. One day while in his study, the Nobel Prize-winning physiologist watched lightning slice the sky. A loud clap of thunder followed every flash of light. Hess noted that almost any observant bystander would quickly recognize that the two phenomena were related. The difference for a scientist, he thought, was the greater number of similar observations necessary to draw a firm conclusion.

His scientific territory, however, was more controversial than the weather. Using electricity, Hess explored the brain and mind. The observations he made and the conclusions that he drew from his own research created a storm of dissent.

At the time, in the first quarter of the twentieth century, electrical stimulation had been limited to the surface of the brain. Hess devised a method for penetrating deep brain structures. Guiding fine wires through holes in a cat's skull, the doctor carefully inserted them into specific sites just above the upper section of the brainstem. He attached cables to the electrodes and, when the anesthetic wore off, sent a gentle electrical current through the electrodes.

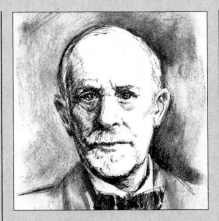

The cat's sudden changes in behavior startled him. A tiny surge of electricity to the cat's hypothalamus, a part of the limbic system, turned the gentle animal into a ferocious beast. It hissed and snarled, arched its back, bristled its fur and lashed its tail as though mortally threatened. Hess reached toward the cat, but it swiftly tried to claw him.

More surprising, Hess found that he could induce varied behavior. Depending on the particular brain site stimulated, the cat would eat, drink, curl up and sleep or become sexually aroused. Hess discovered he could also control the animal's breathing and heartbeat.

The Swiss scientist pursued the theory that he could electrically induce emotions. But his peers quickly denounced the theory. Did the cat's behavior indicate a response to

real anger, or was it sham rage, as his critics charged? They believed that Hess had triggered a series of physical reactions duplicating those of rage, without the felt emotion. Surely, they argued, something so complicated as an emotion could not be recreated by an impersonal surge of electricity.

He had not underestimated the complexity of his subject matter, however. "Only little by little and ever so slowly did the veil lift a bit here and there," Hess wrote. A demanding researcher, he conducted experiments for twenty-five years before publishing his final conclusions. More than 400 cats passed through his laboratory in that time. He stimulated thousands of brain sites, most of them in the hypothalamus, and observed the responses. Hess held firmly to his belief that true emotion could be electrically induced.

In the 1950s, a few years after his monographs were published, other scientists duplicated his experiments and confirmed his theory.

Hess's findings were eventually "well received," he modestly remarked. He was granted the Nobel Prize in 1949. By mapping areas of the living brain never before explored, his technique ushered in a new era of brain research.

Psychologist James Olds accidentally discovered "pleasure centers" in the hypothalamus, while stimulating the brainstems of a group of rats. Each time a rat approached a certain corner of a specially wired box, Olds applied a current transmitted through a wire leash to the animal's head. Most of the rats avoided that corner, but, to the scientist's surprise, one rat kept returning. Later, Olds discovered he had placed the electrode too high in that rat's brain, planting it in the hypothalamus instead of the brainstem.

Further studies confirmed the hypothalamic pleasure centers. Olds put rats in a box where they could press a pedal connected to electrodes in their brains. Each press of the pedal delivered an electrical jolt. Electrodes placed in other regions elicited a few pushes of the pedal. But with electrodes embedded in the hypothalamus, the animals pressed incessantly. Some of them pumped five thousand times an hour, for hours on end. In another test, the rats had to cross an electric grid to reach the pedal. Olds found that even a strong shock did not deter them.

Swiss physiologist Walter Hess, another ESB pioneer, found that stimulating frontal regions of the hypothalamus produced signs of fear in cats. Yet other scientists, stimulating the back of the hypothalamus, propelled animals into frenzy.

Limbic Floodgates

Through connections with the pea-sized pituitary gland, the hypothalamus controls growth and sexual behavior. On orders from the hypothalamus, the pituitary organizes the endocrine glands' release of hormones into the bloodstream. The hypothalamus sends its commands to the pituitary through a mass of nerve fibers called the pituitary stalk. Veins also channel hypothalamic chemicals to other sites in the brain and body.

When sensors in the hypothalamus detect a drop in hormones in the bloodstream, the hypothalamus instructs the pituitary to step up production. It is a delicate system of reciprocity. Through sexual arousal, hormones act directly on the hypothalamus which, in turn, orders the actions of the pituitary. So crucial is it in regulating sexual impulses that injury to certain hypothalamic regions can kill the sex urge entirely.

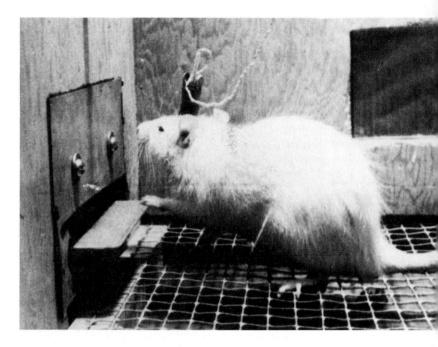

Wearing an electrode for a hat, a wired rat presses a pedal for a split-second electrical jolt. Some tap all day, stimulating hypothalamic areas that produce pleasure. Probing other regions of the hypothalamus provokes rage, fear or the urge to flee.

*In danger or stress the body will
automatically react by releasing
a flood of energizing hormones.
The tiger trainer's survival depends
on his heightened awareness and
attention.*

*On guard against the night, the
hypothalamus commands fight or
flight. Eyes open wider to peer
through the dark, heart beats faster,
fuel and defenses pump more quickly
to muscles anticipating peril.*

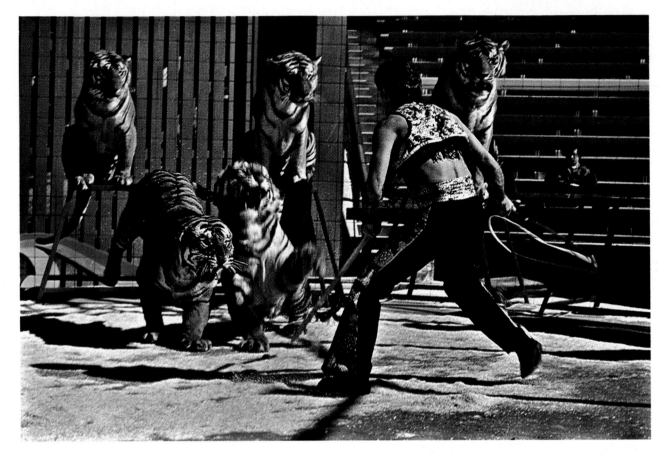

The hypothalamus also coordinates the "fight or flight" reaction, the body's response to the feeling of fear in times of emergency. A commuter stepping off the night train on the way home suddenly spies the silhouette of a figure in the shadows of the subway. Cautiously he makes his way toward the escalator, but on reaching it, the figure darts into the open and blocks his path. The traveler, fearing he is about to be attacked, suffers emotional stress of such magnitude that his body undergoes immediate changes. First to react is the hypothalamus which organizes a chain reaction of defenses with a single aim: to put the body in top physical condition to cope with the emergency.

Its neighbor, the pituitary gland, takes over the command. Tipped off to the danger by hypothalamic chemicals seeping through bridges of blood, the pituitary signals one of its endocrine gates to bolster the defenses. The pituitary flashes the message by secreting a stress hormone known as adrenocorticotropic (ACTH), which finds its way through the bloodstream to the fighting adrenal glands on the kidneys, so-called because in anger or fear they produce even more stress hormones. Another adrenal chemical begins converting fats and proteins into sugar. The adrenals spew out adrenalin and noradrenalin, the heart thumps faster, blood pressure rises and pupils of the eyes dilate wildly to improve vision. The combined surge of hormones relaxes the bronchial tubes for deeper breathing, increases blood sugar to supply maximum energy, slows down the digestive process to conserve muscular energy and shifts blood supplies so they are able to clot more easily on an open wound. In a matter of seconds, the body has become a tight coil of vastly altered substances. Poised to meet the emergency, it can now perform feats of strength and endurance far beyond its normal capacity.

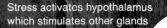
Stress activates hypothalamus
which stimulates other glands

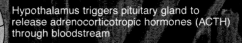
Hypothalamus triggers pituitary gland to
release adrenocorticotropic hormones (ACTH)
through bloodstream

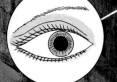
Hair shaft becomes erect

Bronchial tubes open
for deeper breathing

ACTH

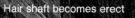
Eye dilates

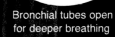
Heart beats faster,
contracts strongly

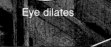
Blood pressure rises

Blood sugar
increases,
digestive system
slows down

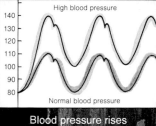
Muscles contract,
blood vessels widen
to allow additional
blood flow

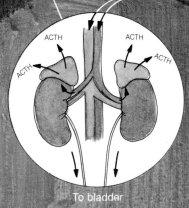
Adrenal glands release
norepinephrine (NE) to
nervous system and
more ACTH to
bloodstream

To bladder

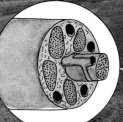
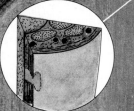
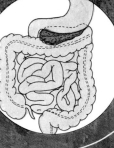
Surface vessels of the skin contract,
causing it to pale; and, if injured,
blood clots more quickly

José Delgado

Engineer of Emotion

Mind control is a popular subject of science fiction. Writer David Rorvik envisions an "electroligarchy" — a society divided into castes, each determined by the number of electrodes individuals have implanted in their brains. The rulers have none; members of the lowest caste have 500. These members "could dig ditches all day and love every minute of it," imagines Rorvik.

Physiologist José Delgado, whose controversial experiments inspired the writer, has been a proponent of electrical stimulation of the brain since the 1940s. He acknowledges that the "possibility of scientific annihilation of personal identity, or even worse, its purposeful control, has sometimes been considered a future threat more awful than atomic holocaust." But, Delgado cautions, "scientific discoveries and technology cannot be shelved because of real or imaginary dangers."

He developed a means to stimulate the brain by remote control, which freed test animals from the cables that had restricted their natural movements in experiments. He implanted electrodes in the brain and attached them to a device — a stimoceiver — worn on the animal's skull or under the skin. The stimo-

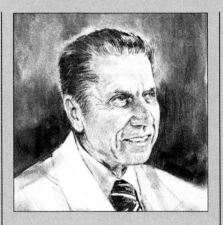

ceiver, directed by an experimenter or computer, picked up and transmitted radio signals through the electrodes.

Delgado used ESB to induce frowning, chewing, walking and other movements in animals. He also stimulated rage or fear and calmed aggressive creatures.

In social situations, control of simple animal behavior created complex consequences. Ali, the bold leader of a monkey colony, was stern, aggressive and feared by his subordinates. When Delgado stimulated a portion of Ali's brain, the monkey's expression subtly changed, and Delgado watched as other members of the colony approached him with seeming confidence.

Delgado gave the monkeys the opportunity to control Ali's behavior. He put a lever inside the cage connected to a

radio transmitter that halted Ali's aggressiveness. A female, often harassed by Ali in the past, quickly learned to press the lever when Ali tried to assert himself. "Peace and war — at least in the monkey colonies — are within the control of the scientist," concluded Delgado.

Delgado would like to use his technique in human society — not as a tool for mass control, but as an educational and medical instrument. With it and other exploratory tools, the scientist argued, man may be able to better understand and better control his brain and emotions, leading to "the education of more sociable and less cruel human beings."

Delgado believes man has spent too much time improving his external world and too little time enhancing the internal world of the mind: "We have reached a critical turning point in the evolution of man at which the mind can be used to influence its own structure, functions and purpose, thereby ensuring both the preservation and advance of civilization."

Delgado realizes his radical ideas will not be readily embraced, but holds that their time will come, as it did for the once controversial use of inoculations and fluoridation.

While some scientists have used ESB to track the brain's emotional pathways, others have experimented with a more controversial application — behavior control. Transistorized radio receivers, activating cranial electrodes, allowed stimulation by remote control. With them, experimenters have tamed fierce monkeys and turned friendly cats into hostile animals. Yale University physiologist José Delgado stopped a charging bull by pressing a transmitter button.

Despite improved technology, explorers probing still virginal territory of the brain cannot predict exactly how stimulation will affect behavior. Two subjects can react differently to stimulation of the same brain site. Scientists have found that individual neuronal circuits are just as unique as fingerprints, making it virtually impossible for scientists to activate the same cluster of nerve cells in different people. Moreover, pleasure and punishment circuits, researchers discovered, appear to lie only fractions of centimeters apart.

Some experimenters have advocated ESB to curb violent behavior, but a mass behavior control program involving entire populations seems improbable. Delgado himself dismisses the prospect as "remote, if not impossible." He admits that "theoretically it would be possible to regulate aggressiveness, productivity or sleep" with brain electrodes, "but this technique requires specialized knowledge, refined skills and a detailed and complex exploration in each individual, because of the existence of anatomical and physiological variability."

The Psychosurgery Controversy

Altering human behavior by surgically destroying brain tissue is far more controversial. Unlike ESB, psychosurgery permanently alters the brain and can profoundly transform an individual's personality. Opponents damn the practice as mutilation of the mind, while advocates claim that psychosurgery is often the last hope for severely disturbed psychiatric patients who do not respond to other kinds of therapy.

In 1935, psychosurgery gained a medical following when Portuguese neurologist Antônio de Egas Moniz became its leading advocate. Inspired by reports that agitated animals became placid

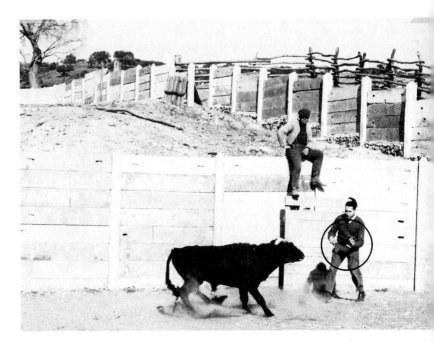

after removal of their prefrontal lobes (an area lying behind the forehead), Moniz wondered if a similar operation could alleviate severe emotional disorders in patients. He devised leucotomy, a technique of drilling holes through the skull and severing fibers that connected the prefrontal lobes with the limbic system. The technique spread rapidly in the next decade, spurred by lack of effective alternative treatments for severe emotional disturbances and by the development of a new technique that removed leucotomy from the exclusive domain of neurosurgery. Developed in 1946 by neurologist Walter Freeman, transorbital lobotomy did not require opening the skull. It could therefore be performed by general practitioners and psychiatrists as well as surgeons. Freeman performed more than three thousand operations by thrusting a sharp, thin instrument through the upper eye socket to sever the nerve fibers of the frontal lobes.

Despite refinements in psychosurgical techniques, the use of lobotomy declined rapidly after 1955. From operations numbering in the tens of thousands, it was clear that lobotomy made patients apathetic, unresponsive or wildly impulsive. Its many physical side effects included poor coordination, epileptic seizures and incontinence.

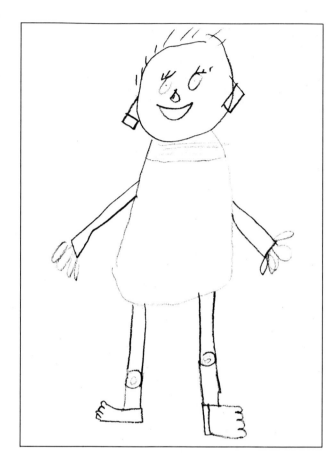 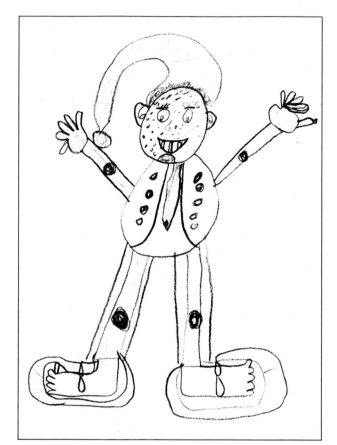

A barefoot figure scrawled by an eight-year-old betrays hyperactivity. After a month's treatment with a drug to stimulate neurotransmitters in the brain, the youngster's concentration improved, enabling him to draw a more detailed figure with the proper number of fingers and toes. Additive-free diet and behavior therapy in the classroom offer other means of controlling hyperactivity disorders.

With the benefit of hindsight, both the medical and lay worlds are overwhelmingly opposed to indiscriminate psychosurgery. It is only performed on several hundred psychiatric patients each year in the United States.

Seeking Chemical Cures

Even before lobotomy fell out of favor, scientists had begun to suspect that chemical imbalances in the brain might be the cause of some forms of mental illness. First introduced in 1952, drugs known as major tranquilizers have become the primary treatment for victims of severe mental illness. Chlorpromazine, manufactured as an antihistamine, was found to be an effective sedative. Psychiatrists soon began testing its calming effects on schizophrenics. The drug not only calmed patients but relieved the schizophrenic symptoms of disordered thoughts and hallucinations. Only within the last decade have scientists begun to understand how chlorpromazine and newer antischizophrenic drugs work. These medications seem to reverse a suspected surplus of the neurotransmitter dopamine, probably by blocking receptors, or nerve-cell sites, in the brain that bind to dopamine.

The first antidepressant drug, iproniazid, was also a serendipitous discovery. First used to treat tuberculosis, the drug so excited patients that doctors stopped prescribing it. But its mood-lifting properties made it an excellent possibility for the treatment of depression. Iproniazid works chemically by blocking the enzyme monoamine oxidase, a neurotransmitter thought to be produced during intense emotional states. Used widely during the late 1950s, iproniazid and related drugs are now rarely given because of adverse side effects. More commonly prescribed are lithium for manic depression and tricyclics for depression. Tricyclics are thought to lift depression by increasing levels of the neurotransmitters norepinephrine and serotonin. The discovery of these drugs has been hailed as a psychiatric milestone, enabling thousands of schizophrenics to live away from mental institutions.

Doctors also use drugs to treat hyperactivity. As many as 13 percent of all school-age children in the United States may suffer from its symp-toms: excessive moodiness, short attention spans, agitation and unpredictable behavior. Many researchers suspect hyperactives have deficient neurotransmitter levels. Two Yale scientists who examined the spinal fluid of hyperactive children found an insufficiency of dopamine. Amphetamines and other stimulants have the paradoxical effect of calming these children, probably by increasing neurotransmitter levels.

The Sexual Brain

As scientists gain more insight into the physiological underpinnings of behavior, a question which for decades has been the topic of heated debate in academic circles has been brought into sharper focus: Is heredity or environment the predominant force in shaping human behavior? While few scientists would deny that both are crucial elements, recent studies appear to give the edge to the former in sexual behavior.

Until recently, many scientists thought that an individual's sexual identity and behavior were determined more by social attitudes and upbringing than by heredity. Johns Hopkins psychologist John Money and colleagues summed up the prevailing view of the 1960s, saying that sexual behavior was not in the genes: "Psychologically, sexuality . . . becomes differentiated as masculine or feminine in the course . . . of growing up."

Mounting evidence that male and female animal brains are chemically and structurally different has led to a reversal of this concept. Many researchers now suspect that human sexual behavior is the outcome of sex hormones acting on the brain during a critical period before birth. Sex hormones injected into fetal or newborn laboratory animals make them adopt behaviors typical of the opposite sex: A female rat given the male sex hormone testosterone shortly after birth does not ovulate or show female mating behavior; an adult male deprived of male hormones by castration assumes the female mating posture when injected with estrogen, a female sex hormone.

Evidence that the activity of sex hormones during fetal life determines human sexuality comes from a study of thirty-eight children in the Dominican Republic. The children were born with ill-defined genitals. Many of them were raised as girls. Their lives changed at puberty when male characteristics suddenly emerged: deepened voices, muscle development and male genitals. As adults, they have lived as normal males, all but two weathering the transition with ease. Scientists later found that the children had been victims of a genetic disease which retarded the metabolism of testosterone until puberty, at which time the sudden surge of male hormones abruptly masculinized them. Cornell University endocrinologist Julianne Imperato-McGinley, who conducted the study, concluded, "The sex of rearing could not have been the predominant force in shaping their sexual identity."

In 1973, a British study confirmed that the brains of male and female laboratory rats are chemically different. The scientists found differences in the distribution of nerve connections in the preoptic region — an area next to the hypothalamus thought to be related to reproduction. UCLA researchers also discovered structural differences in this region; one cell cluster was five times larger in the male than in the female rat. Manipulating hormone levels shrinks this cell cluster in males and expands it in females.

Scientists have not been able to confirm that such differences also exist in the human brain, but studies of patients with brain damage and findings from psychological and behavioral tests suggest that the female brain is organized differently from the male brain. The female brain seems to be more adroit at switching between left and right hemispheres. While this flexibility bestows greater verbal skills, it might be a drawback in mathematical, visual and conceptual thinking — activities in which the more narrowly focused male brain is thought to excel. Researchers Karl Pribram and Diane McGuinness sum up this theory from the perspective that "men and women are *different*. What needs to be made equal is the value placed upon these differences."

Selfish Genes?

A new discipline called sociobiology theorizes that much animal and human social behavior springs from a biological base. According to this theory, many behavior patterns are innate, programmed into each individual's genes for the sole purpose of bolstering the prospects of survival. Led by a group of American and British biologists and zoologists, sociobiologists see themselves as heirs of Charles Darwin, completing his theory of evolution. In the nineteenth century, Darwin argued that all organisms evolve by a process called natural selection. Those better able to adapt to their environment survive and reproduce; the remainder die out. Sociobiologists go even further, maintaining that only the behavior patterns which promote the genes' survival are passed on. The organism does not exist for itself; its purpose is to reproduce genes and to serve as their temporary carrier.

The crux of sociobiological theory is its bold explanation for altruism. Programmed to behave in a manner that ensures survival of his genes, an individual performs acts of kindness for selfish reasons — making sacrifices for relatives because they carry the same genes and helping non-relatives with expectations of reciprocal favors.

Sexual behavior, according to sociobiologists, also ensures survival of the genes. Machismo is a strategy for winning a female mate, who supposedly responds to bravado as evidence of good genes. In the sociobiological perspective, women are at a genetic disadvantage because, with a heavier investment in their offspring and more limited reproductive capability, they have far fewer chances to spread their genes.

Since the 1975 publication of *Sociobiology*, by Harvard University zoologist Edward O. Wilson, sociobiology has divided college faculties and raised the specter of racist, sexist and elitist attitudes. Many also object to its implication that man is devoid of free will, a mere slave to the selfish ambitions of biology and genes.

But within sociobiology's doctrines, there is a glimmer of hope. Oxford University zoologist Richard Dawkins believes that "even if we look on the dark side and assume that individual man is fundamentally selfish, our conscious foresight — our capacity to simulate the future in imagination — could save us from the worst selfish excesses. . . . We have at least the mental equipment to foster our long-term selfish interest. . . . We have the power to defy the selfish genes of our birth."

Photomicrographs of brain sections from a bird show the dark region concerned with courtship song much larger in a male zebra finch, top, than in a female, below. That explains why the males sing and their mates do not. Scientists suspect that sexual differences also exist in the human brain. Men and women seem to have differently organized brains, but structural proof is yet to come.

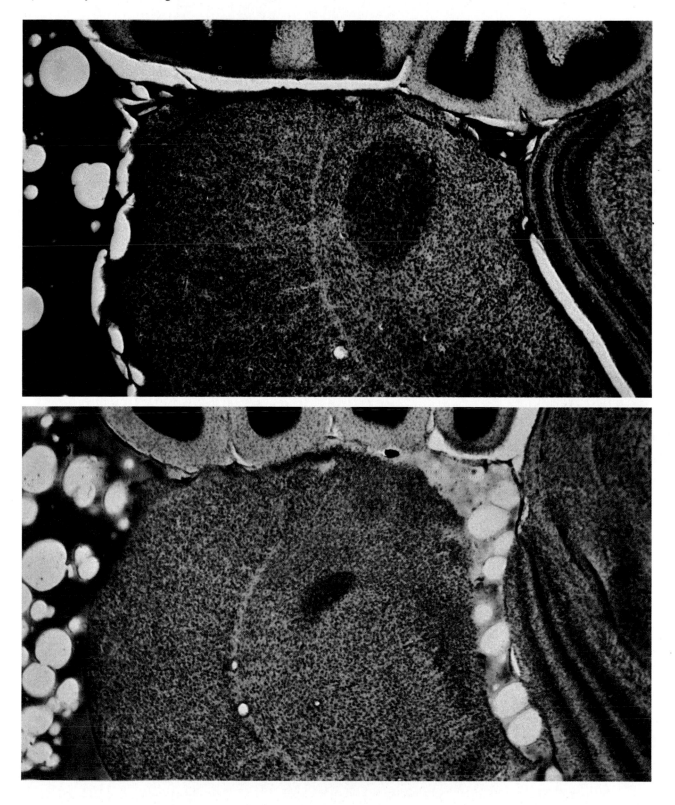

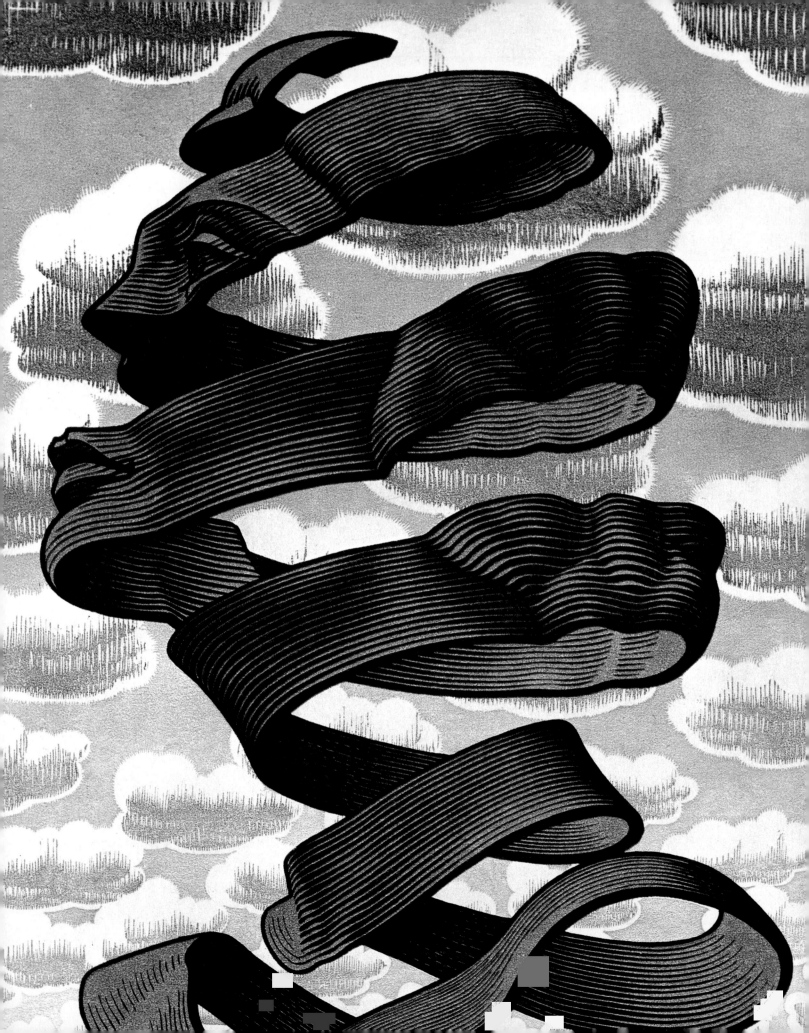

Chapter 8

Mazes of the Mind

In the fall of 1880, one of Austria's most prominent physicians, Dr. Josef Breuer, was summoned to help an ailing young woman named Bertha Pappenheim. Suffering from exhaustion and a persistent, ominous cough, she lay bedridden in the home where her father was slowly dying from tuberculosis.

After examining Bertha, Breuer found that she suffered not from a lung disease but from a nervous disorder. Her cough was only one of many bewildering symptoms, including hallucinations, poor vision, partial paralysis and an apparent difficulty in hearing. Breuer diagnosed hysteria, a perplexing disease that many doctors of his day dismissed. In medical circles, hysteria was viewed as deception by attention-hungry patients. The usual treatment was hypnotic trance in which the doctor told his patient to give up the symptoms. Many patients did, if only temporarily.

In Bertha's case, however, Breuer decided to take a different approach. When he hypnotized her, instead of suggesting that she abandon her symptoms, he asked what troubled her, why was she so distressed. In posing this question, Breuer had opened the door to Bertha's tormented mind, taking an important first step down the path toward understanding the mazes of the human mind. It would prove to be an exhilarating yet terrifying journey, and one from which Breuer himself eventually recoiled.

Over the course of more than a year, Breuer helped Bertha remember and relive some of the most painful moments of her past, and in doing so, freed her of their tormenting power. Together, physician and patient invented the "talking cure," as Bertha called it. Breuer mentioned this woman — later known as the famous "Anna O." — to a young friend and colleague named Sigmund Freud. That day, November 18, 1882, Freud would later remember as his first awareness of the immense power of the unconscious.

The human brain holds the unconscious, source of our individual drives, our uniqueness. We search its mazes, as insubstantial as the airy clouds amidst the womanly head in M. C. Escher's wood engraving, Rind, *to find personality.*

Freud's interest in hypnosis sent him to Paris to study under the famous French neurologist Jean Martin Charcot. His own research into nervous disorders, Breuer's "talking cure," the memories, fears and desires of the patients Freud and Breuer subsequently treated — these are the seeds from which modern psychoanalysis sprouted. With this new method of studying the mind grew a new view of the mind, a new notion of man and a modern legend that would influence every aspect of Western society.

The Unconscious Surfacing

Freud's work with hysteria convinced him that the keys to his patients' suffering lay buried within their own minds, but that the causes were mostly beyond their conscious reach. A poor hypnotist, Freud searched for a new method to gain access to the unconscious — the name he gave that portion of the mind lying outside conscious awareness. He developed "free association," a technique in which he would sit beyond sight of his patient and suggest subjects for discussion, then allow the patient to say whatever came to mind. Freud sifted through these ramblings in search of ideas that might be relevant to the patient's problem.

Free association led Freud to psychoanalysis, his revolutionary explanation for the workings of the human mind. This theory was based on two underlying principles. First, that most of the psychic energy an individual possesses is used up by the unconscious, not the conscious, mind; second, that all actions are determined by childhood events. The object of free association was to trace the thread of unrestrained thought back to the initiating event whose memory lay buried within the unconscious. If the psychoanalyst could piece together these threads from the past, the patient could understand his behavior and be cured.

Although free association, dream interpretation and other techniques for probing the unconscious gained him much recognition, it was Freud's explanation of the origin and function of the unconscious that brought him world fame.

Intrigued by the depths to which his patients buried their sexual fantasies, Freud came to believe that sexuality underlies much behavior and that sexual conflicts are the cause of most personality disorders. Freud scandalized society with his views on sexuality, in which he placed the libido, or sexual energy, as the primary force which drives each individual.

Equally controversial was his theory of infantile sexual development. Freud believed that personality developed from an individual's experience in passing through five stages, each determined by the child's interest in a specific bodily zone. These were the oral, anal, phallic, latent and genital stages. If a child encountered a problem at any of these stages, he would become fixated there and expend more energy in activities connected with that stage. An oral fixation could cause excessive indulgence in oral activities, while fixation at the anal stage could lead to an overemphasis on personal hygiene.

Freud's famed Oedipal complex arises from the phallic stage, when interest focuses on the genitals. Freud felt the Greek myth of a boy who grew up to marry his mother and kill his father symbolized a universal pattern of human behavior. At this stage, children develop an attraction to the parent of the opposite sex.

In the latency stage, which follows the phallic one, sexual impulses are dormant. The child turns his energy to mastering skills needed for living in the external world. In the next period, the genital stage, the adolescent shifts his sexual focus to others and begins mature sexuality.

In explaining how the unconscious dealt with powerful basic drives, Freud created an entire universe within the hidden mind. He called the expression of the sex drive and other biological urges the id.

Psychic Struggle

Constantly seeking pleasure and lacking regard for consequences, the id has been suppressed by the larger forces of human society. In Freud's theory, two other aspects of personality grow out of the id. The ego, the perceived self, is the part of the personality that deals with reality. Its role is to bring the impulsive id into line with the demands of the real world. It also hones the mind's powers of judgment and planning. The superego, the second element, is the conscience

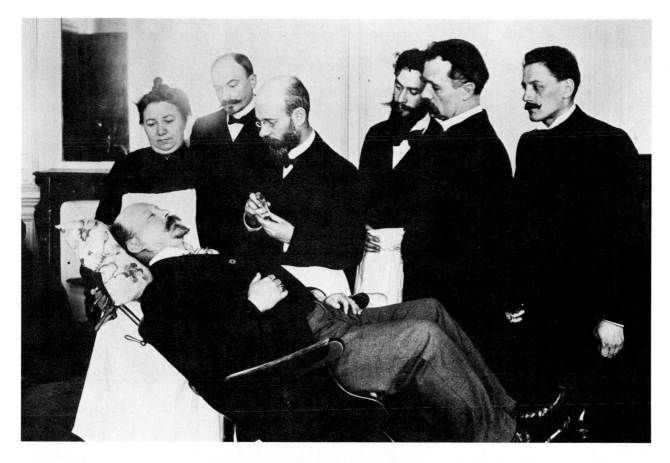

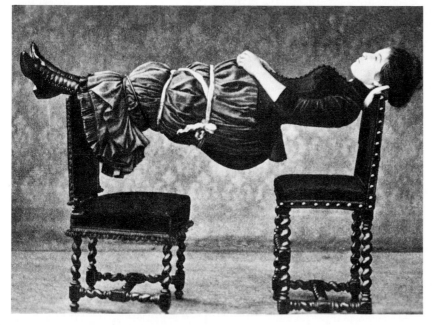

In the dreamlike trance of hypnosis, the brain and body tap powers and thoughts beyond reach of the conscious mind. Early physiologists believed hypnosis was a path to the unconscious. Several watch a colleague ease his patient into a trance, above. Others saw only parlor entertainment in the strange state of mind that could elicit from a prim Victorian lady, left, a feat of strength she would never attempt while awake.

Freudians believe personality has three sides. The superego on the left strives for moral perfection. Yet on the right, the id—the mainspring of our passions and drives—demands pleasure at any cost. The logical ego is caught between these two extremes and tries to balance them. Personality is really a constant tug-of-war between these three elements, each one trying to become the dominant power.

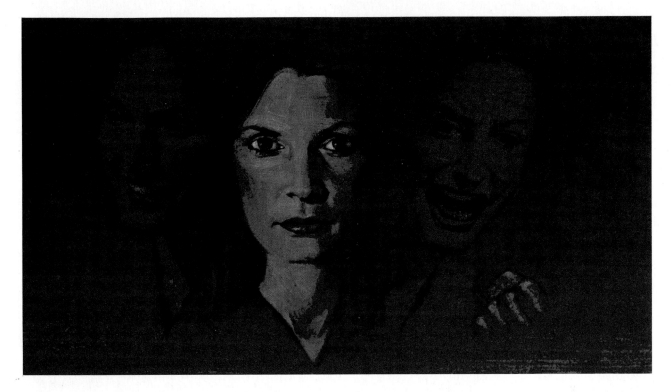

which tries to impose moral values on both the id and the ego. The superego is both inborn and acquired by the child as he internalizes the values instilled in him by his parents.

When the impulses of the id collide with the realistic demands of the ego or the moral strictures of the superego — or if they join forces with one against the other — the result is intolerable conflict. If unresolved, this conflict can lead to anxiety, neurotic symptoms or psychosis — the most severe mental disorder.

Freud's theories of personality and the unconscious loosed a storm of controversy. His belief that every person is driven by powerful, even perverse, sexual drives barely under control sent shock waves across Victorian Europe and then to America. His theory of infantile sexuality offended many. But even as his disciples left him to pursue their own psychological theories, Freud's influence over twentieth-century morality and culture grew deeper. He took psychology out of the clinic, and through his essays on wit, humor and dreams, brought to the public fascinating explanations of their everyday behavior.

Attracted by Freud's daring theories, some of his disciples became influential theorists in their own right. Psychologist Alfred Adler worked with Freud for nearly ten years. He agreed with the use of dreams and free association in the analysis of personality. But while Freud concentrated on the sources of conflicts, Adler was intrigued by their forms. Believing Freud overemphasized biological drives, he theorized that self-generated goals and social relationships developed personality. Adler thought the first experience of life was the helplessness of infancy, which led to a sense of inferiority. He saw the motivating force behind personality and behavior as a perpetual struggle for power.

Swiss psychiatrist Carl Gustav Jung, another distinguished follower, realized that many of Freud's theories mirrored his own. Of their first meeting, Jung later recalled, "What he said about his sexual theory impressed me. Nevertheless, his words could not remove my hesitations and doubts. I tried to advance these reservations of mine on several occasions, but each time he would attribute them to my lack of experience."

Sigmund Freud

The Father of Psychoanalysis

"I have found my tyrant and in his service I know no limits. My tyrant is psychology." Through his tyrant, Sigmund Freud revolutionized the study of the mind. His reach went far beyond the limits of science. Freud changed the way mankind viewed the mind, human motivations and behavior.

Freud began his dynamic career halfheartedly. He had wanted to be a research scientist, but a teacher advised Freud to take up the more lucrative practice of medicine, a task he did not relish.

In 1886, the young Viennese doctor, intending to specialize in neurological disorders, opened a private practice in his home. Many of his patients were hysterical women suffering from mysterious disorders that had no physiological sources. Freud was fascinated by their uneasy minds. His exploratory techniques for treating them and the theories he developed from this work became psychoanalysis, his key to the unconscious.

As his knowledge of the powers and provinces of the mind expanded, Freud kept to himself, only maintaining close ties with his family and a few friends. Soon after his father died in 1896, Freud's isolation increased. Distraught and doubting his own theories,

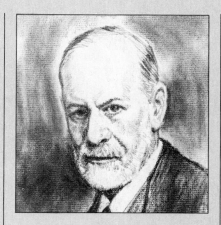

Freud began a painstaking process of self-analysis. He felt he was "in a cocoon, and God knows what kind of beast will creep out of it." His work from this turbulent period was his greatest. In *The Interpretation of Dreams*, published in 1900, he portrayed dreams as a wellspring of unconscious thought and presented the Oedipus complex, one of his controversial theories of childhood sexual development.

Warmed by the international attention his book earned, Freud sought out others with similar interests and formed the Vienna Psycho-Analytical Society. By 1908, the society had twenty-two members, including Freud's most famous followers, Alfred Adler and Carl Jung. Freud was the established father of the group, but Adler and Jung were not ideal sons. Their theories led

them away from Freud's and attracted other members who followed in their wake. Freud viewed their departure with bitterness. "So we are at last rid of them," he wrote to a remaining member, "the brutal sanctimonious Jung and his disciples."

The framework supporting Freud's theories, an intricate model of the mind, developed throughout most of his career. His final concept, appearing in *The Ego and the Id* in 1923, divided the mind into three components. The id, ego and superego compromised in the human psyche.

Freud once professed his best work was done when he suffered a "moderate amount of misery." The last years of his life were not easy ones. He underwent painful operations to treat cancer of the jaw, yet he continued his work. With equal determination, he refused to leave Vienna during the Nazi invasion of 1938. Only when they arrested his daughter Anna was the frail eighty-one-year-old man persuaded to flee for safety.

Freud questioned how the future would judge his work. "Scientific research and doubt are inseparable," he wrote, "and I have surely not discovered more than a small fragment of truth."

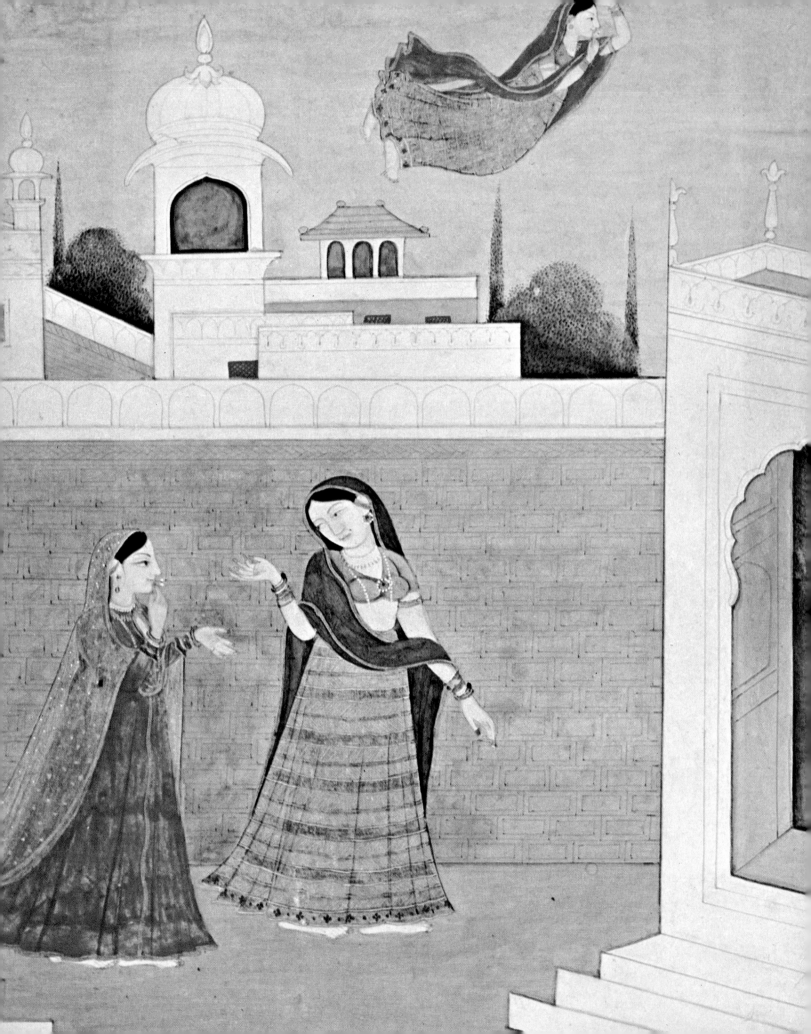

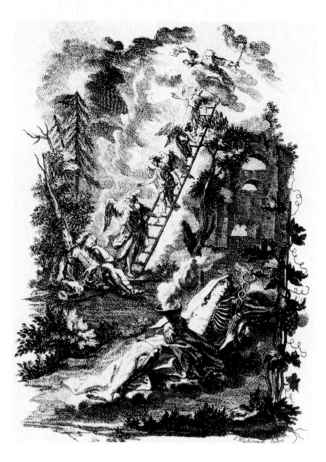

"And he dreamed, and behold a ladder . . . reached to heaven," records Genesis in its account of Jacob's dream. Dreams were important events in the Bible. The eighteenth-century engraving, above, personifies his dream in a figure half flesh, half skeleton, reflecting the ancient view that sleep is akin to death. While Jacob's ladder gave access to God, angelic flight served Usha, mythical maiden of India. The nineteenth-century print, opposite, shows her soaring serenely in a dream common to the sleeping visions of most mankind. But is its meaning the same for all? Carl Jung thought not; experts still debate the question.

Beginning in 1912, with the publication of a major work, *Psychology of the Unconscious,* Jung's views came into open conflict with Freud's and thus the two men parted along their theoretical paths.

Jung viewed the unconscious as an important, functioning part of the human mind, full of the mysteries that give life richness, color and depth. As a child he had precocious insight into the nature of his "two personalities" — one a worldly scholar, the other an introspective seeker. They alternately dominated his consciousness, one leading, the other not far behind. Jung kept his personal revelations to himself. "My entire youth can be understood in terms of this secret," he recalled at age eighty-three. "It induced in me an almost unendurable loneliness."

Dream's Riches

He thought the unconscious communicated to the conscious mind through symbolic images that appeared in dreams as analogies and parables. Freud used his patients' dreams as a departure into other subjects through free association. Jung thought "this was a misleading and inadequate use of the rich fantasies that the unconscious produces in sleep. . . . Very often dreams have a definite, evidently purposeful structure, indicating an underlying idea of intention. . . . I therefore began to consider whether one should pay more attention to the actual form and content of a dream." He considered this "a turning point in the development of my psychology."

Jung believed in the "collective unconscious," psychic information common to all mankind, which he divided into archetypes. The archetypes were inherited, empty forms that became filled by the individual's perceptions of the world. Jung named one archetype "The Mother." This image, based on myth, became personalized by experience with one's own mother. The "personal unconscious" was the individual's storehouse for information once conscious, but later repressed. In dreams, the personal unconscious appeared as an alter ego, a second self, denied conscious freedom by the idealistic ego. Jung thought that although certain motifs could recur — like running and falling — dream symbols were expressions of individual experiences.

Behaviorism's school of thought holds that "reinforcement" through reward or punishment is the key to all learning, for pigeons and humans as well. Below, laboratory pigeons Jack and Jill communicate

with symbols to get food. "What color?" asks Jack. Jill peeks and tells. Jack's "Thank you" dispenses her food pellet. He then pecks the key for the color she had seen to reward himself with a pellet, too.

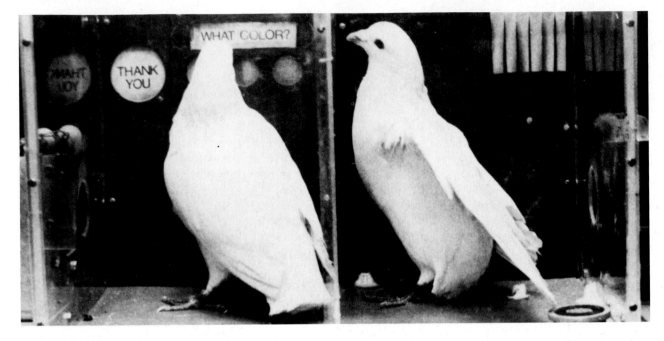

Although Adler and Jung greatly expanded Freud's original theories of the unconscious, they remained in agreement with his fundamental three-part psychic structure. The next generation of psychologists sought to move away from Freud's deterministic psychology which left little of man's behavior to free will. They differ with Freud's interpretation of the ego as guardian of the id. Known as ego psychologists, they believe instead that the ego has functions of its own in perception, motor functioning and problem solving. Influential ego psychologist Erik Erikson believes that personality develops from the resolution or nonresolution of crises occurring through all stages of social development, and that personality continues to grow into old age.

The Science of Behavior

In the early 1900s, as Freud's theories gained momentum, the seeds to another major branch of psychology were sown. Russian physiologist Ivan Pavlov, while researching the digestive system, discovered that he could directly influence an animal's involuntary behavior. By sounding a tone each time a dog was fed, Pavlov "conditioned" the dog to salivate at the sound of the tone, whether or not food was present.

American psychologist John B. Watson applied Pavlov's idea of learned responses to human behavior. In 1913, he wrote, "Psychology, as the behaviorist views it, is a purely objective, experimental branch of natural science which needs introspection as little as do the sciences of chemistry and physics." To prove his theory, Watson presented a young boy with a white rat. As the boy eagerly reached forward, Watson struck an iron bar with a hammer, producing a loud, unpleasant noise. The boy leaped back and broke into tears. After this incident was repeated a number of times, the boy cried merely at the sight of the rat. Watson tested the strength of this learned behavior by exposing the boy to similar items, finding that anything with a furry appearance produced the same results, even a fur coat and a bearded Santa Claus mask.

Perhaps the most controversial behaviorist is Harvard psychologist B. F. Skinner. Developing the "Skinner box," he sought to duplicate in the laboratory the ordinary conditions in which an animal learns. The box contained a tray for food and water, a light, a lever and a window. If a rat pressed the lever, a food pellet dropped into the tray. Gradually, through repetition, the rat learned to press the lever when it wanted to eat.

B. F. Skinner

Exploring the Science of Behavior

"Nothing is worth doing. But we have the instinct to do, and we should be wise enough to do the thing which is most nearly worth doing." When behaviorist B. F. Skinner wrote this rueful pronouncement in 1927, he was one year out of college, and thought writing a worthy career. But he soon realized that he could not write unless he understood behavior. Angrily, he abandoned writing and turned to psychology.

As a student, he spent hours watching squirrels play. He dangled peanuts from strings, tied the strings to branches and watched how the squirrels retrieved the nuts. Later, as a Research Fellow at Harvard University, he developed the Skinner box, a largely automated device that permitted him to study how animals learned. From this work, he drew the conclusion that behavior could only be determined by interaction with the environment. He called any behavior-shaping event "reinforcement," which was either positive or negative.

In 1938, Skinner published the results of his studies in *The Behavior of Organisms.* His first and, perhaps, most influential book, it helped establish behaviorism as a legitimate branch of psychology. By dismissing all but the observable,

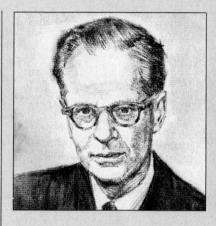

Skinner believed he had introduced scientific objectivity to psychology.

A lover of gadgets, Skinner also constructed the "baby-tender," an enclosed crib with a large glass window, sound-absorbing walls and a climate control system. A 1945 magazine picture of the Skinners at home, with their daughter Debbie in the crib, caused a stir of controversy. Hundreds of parents wrote to Skinner requesting building plans for the crib. But others accused him of being a crackpot who caged his daughter like an animal. "It was natural to suppose," Skinner acknowledged, "that we were experimenting on our daughter as if she were a rat or pigeon."

With the publication of *Walden Two* in 1948, Skinner found success as a writer of fiction, imagining a Utopian society based on his principles of behavior control. The society used positive reinforcement to create the social order; punishment, force or threat did not exist. Competition, aggression and social rank disappeared. Inspired by this fictional world, several organizations established new communities using Skinner's principles. One such society, Twin Oaks in Louisa, Virginia, has existed since 1967.

Skinner's ideas reached a provocative zenith in his 1971 book, *Beyond Freedom and Dignity,* which expanded the assumption beneath his conclusions on all behavior. There is no true free will, he argued. A person who appeared to behave freely was simply free from negative reinforcement. Man's behavior was always under some form of control. If man accepted this idea, Skinner claimed, he would be able to use it to his benefit.

By expanding his theories to include man, Skinner invited much criticism. The jump from rats and pigeons to man was too great, critics charged. Many also reacted indignantly to the theory of behavior control. Skinner, however, saw it not as an ominous shadow, but as a sign of hope: "We have not yet seen," he wrote, "what man can make of man."

Skinner called such patterns of reward "reinforcement." One night, the pellet-dispensing mechanism jammed, so the rat was not rewarded with food. The scientist noticed the result was "extinction," of the learned response.

Skinner varied the patterns of reward. Random rewards that more closely approximated life's experiences still made the rats frequently press the lever. He found such learned behavior more resistant to extinction than any other. One psychologist likened reinforcement to gambling with a slot machine, with the players winning enough to try their luck over and over again.

Skinner theorized that all complex behavior patterns were chains of simpler learned behaviors linked together. He taught pigeons a series of specific responses, which gradually enabled them to play Ping Pong by rolling a ball back and forth across a table. Ping Pong-playing pigeons might seem the stuff of circuses, but Skinner believed they dramatized his theories.

Behavior therapists apply these theories to mankind. Personality, according to behaviorists, develops with the combination of the genetic equipment man inherits and the types of learning to which he is later exposed. Behavior therapy assumes that most abnormal behavior has been learned and can, therefore, be unlearned. This type of therapy has proved most effective in curing phobias, or illogical fears. Watson's study of the boy conditioned to fear furry objects is an example of such a technique in reverse.

Altering Behavior

To treat a child who fears dogs, a behaviorist might give the child a bowl of ice cream and lead a puppy into a corner of the room. The pairing of the feared animal with something enjoyable would be repeated, each time bringing the dog nearer the child. Eventually, a larger dog might be introduced, or more than one. If successful, the treatment would cure the child's fear of dogs.

Behavior therapy treats only the symptoms, critics believe, rather than the sickness. They also argue that, by excluding all of man's inner life, behaviorism greatly oversimplifies human nature. Although completely divergent in theory, psychoanalysis, its offshoots and behaviorism do

have one characteristic in common: the belief that man's personality and behavior are determined by events that shape the mind and mold the responses. To some extent, man therefore appears to be at the mercy of his past experiences and the emotions attached to them.

New Goals, New Values

A major new approach to psychology developed in the 1940s, from the work of Carl C. Rogers, a University of Chicago psychologist. Known as humanistic psychology, it holds that behavioristic formulas and Freudian development stages are offensive to human dignity and individuality. Humanists do not believe in labeling personality and behavior for the sake of theory. They believe that people have the capacity to change and grow throughout life. It is self-awareness that differentiates men from animals. Man alone can choose what to make of his life. Personality and destiny are controlled by each individual.

The goal of humanistic therapy, which Rogers calls "client-centered therapy," is to create a positive environment for the patient by restoring good feelings about himself. The patient can then change his goals to achieve "self-actualization," the realization and fulfillment of his capabilities.

The same goals that structured humanistic psychology have spawned many popular contemporary approaches to therapy. There are now more than 250 therapies practiced. Among the most popular or distinctive therapies are transactional analysis, rebirthing, primal therapy and encounter groups.

Transactional analysis, commonly called TA, is a simplified version of Freudian psychoanalysis. In TA therapy, the id, ego and superego convert to the "child," "adult" and "parent." Patients are taught to see their actions, thoughts and feelings stemming from the interaction of these elements within themselves and others. TA group leaders teach members to recognize when the child within them is talking to the adult in someone else, or when the adult within is responding to the inner parent of another group member.

Rebirthing is another modern therapy that can trace its roots to Freud, although less directly. Freud recognized birth as a potentially traumatic

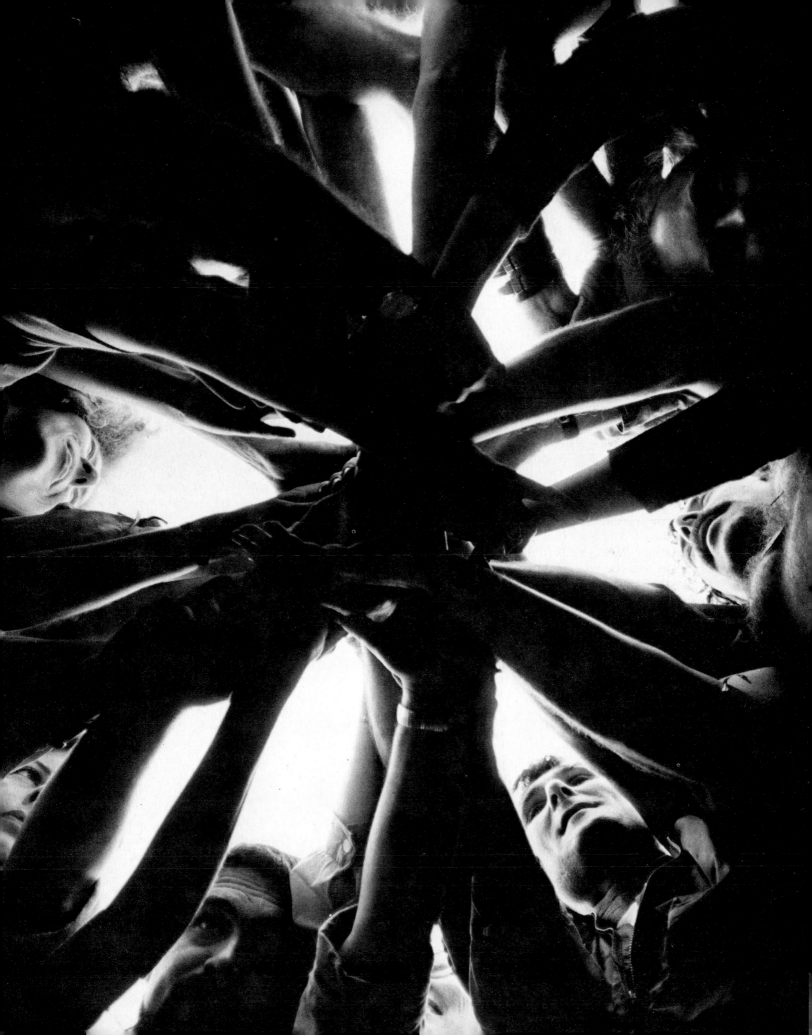

experience. He never actively incorporated the idea into his theories, but one of his early followers, psychotherapist Otto Rank, did. Rank considered birth trauma the common basis of neuroses, or mental disorders stemming from anxiety. "Rebirthers" claim the trauma experienced at birth can be confronted and erased by reenactment, usually while submerged in a tub of water heated to body temperature.

Primal therapy agitates a patient until he erupts with a "primal scream." The founder of primal therapy, California psychologist Arthur Janov, claims that man continually develops an expanding backlog of pain. In defense, the individual develops shields which ultimately interfere with his ability to function normally. Janov's method of therapy encourages a patient to summon up his pain until he is overwhelmed by it, whereupon he screams out, releasing its tension. Once unburdened of this emotional ballast, the patient should be free and healthy.

Encounter group therapies vary, but all stress the importance of understanding one's feelings. To do so, encounter groups try to establish situations which will permit the arousal of new feelings or the examination of troublesome old ones. Group interaction, even if hostile, is encouraged. This interaction may be verbal — from consoling to name calling — and physical — from stroking to punching. Before, during or after such sessions, the group members are asked to discuss their feelings. Group therapy seeks to engender an atmosphere of shared problems, encouraging freer expression of emotion.

A Troubling Reappraisal

A number of recent studies offer pessimistic conclusions about therapy. Different forms of therapy seem to provide no discernible difference in success of treatment. Furthermore, the length of treatment and the experience of the therapist seem to make no measurable difference. An outspoken critic within the profession of psychology, Thomas Szasz, feels "psychotherapy is simply a name we give to two people talking to each other. It's like 'holy' water — it's just water. It doesn't exist unless you believe in it. . . . It is the believing that brings help."

Such ambivalence was underscored by an experiment several years ago in which Stanford psychiatrist D. L. Rosenhan asked healthy subjects to enter mental hospitals across the nation. They were admitted by mimicking classically accepted symptoms of schizophrenia, a severe form of mental illness characterized by disturbances of thought and distortion of reality. Once there, they behaved normally as instructed, but their words and actions were consistently interpreted as schizophrenic by the staff.

The rising use of drugs in the treatment of the mentally ill has also stirred the reappraisal of psychotherapy. Over the last several decades, the number of people in the United States who have mental illnesses requiring treatment has increased nearly three times. But only half as many people are being hospitalized for illnesses — a statistic attributed almost solely to the prescription of drugs.

When drugs proved effective in quelling schizophrenic symptoms, scientists were confronted with a provocative question. Could abnormal behavior be caused by a chemical imbalance in the brain? Studies have indicated that schizophrenics produce too much dopamine, one of dozens of chemicals the brain uses to transmit messages between nerve cells. Drugs that block dopamine help restore the proper balance of chemicals and, by causing schizophrenic symptoms to lessen or disappear, enable schizophrenics to lead nearly normal lives.

The use of drugs alone in treating mental illness has drawn much the same criticism as behavior therapy — drugs treat only the symptoms, not the illness. Surveys conducted at the Western Psychiatric Institute of Pittsburgh showed that schizophrenic patients treated with both psychotherapy and drugs were less likely to suffer a relapse than patients treated solely with psychotherapy or drugs. Although traditional Freudian psychoanalysts are among the members of the profession most inclined to disapprove of the use of drugs in treating disorders of the mind, Freud himself believed that drugs might one day be useful in treating mental illness: "The future may teach us how to exercise a direct influence by particular chemical substances."

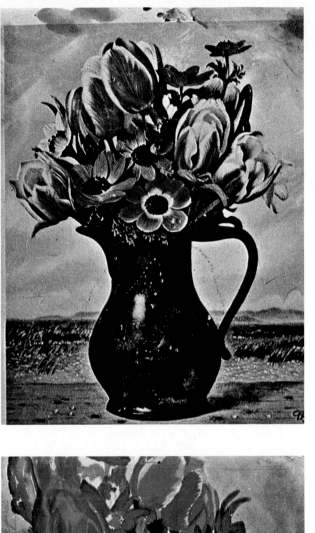

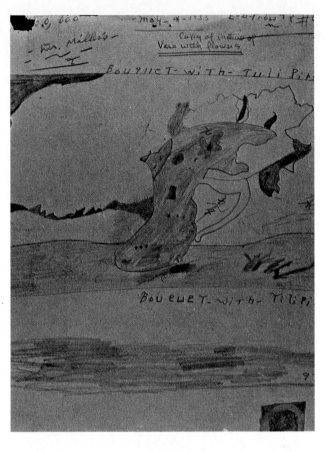

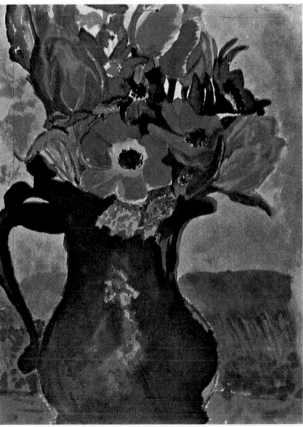

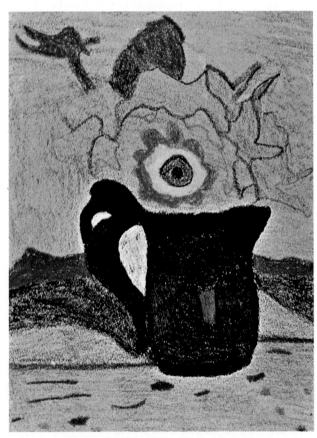

119

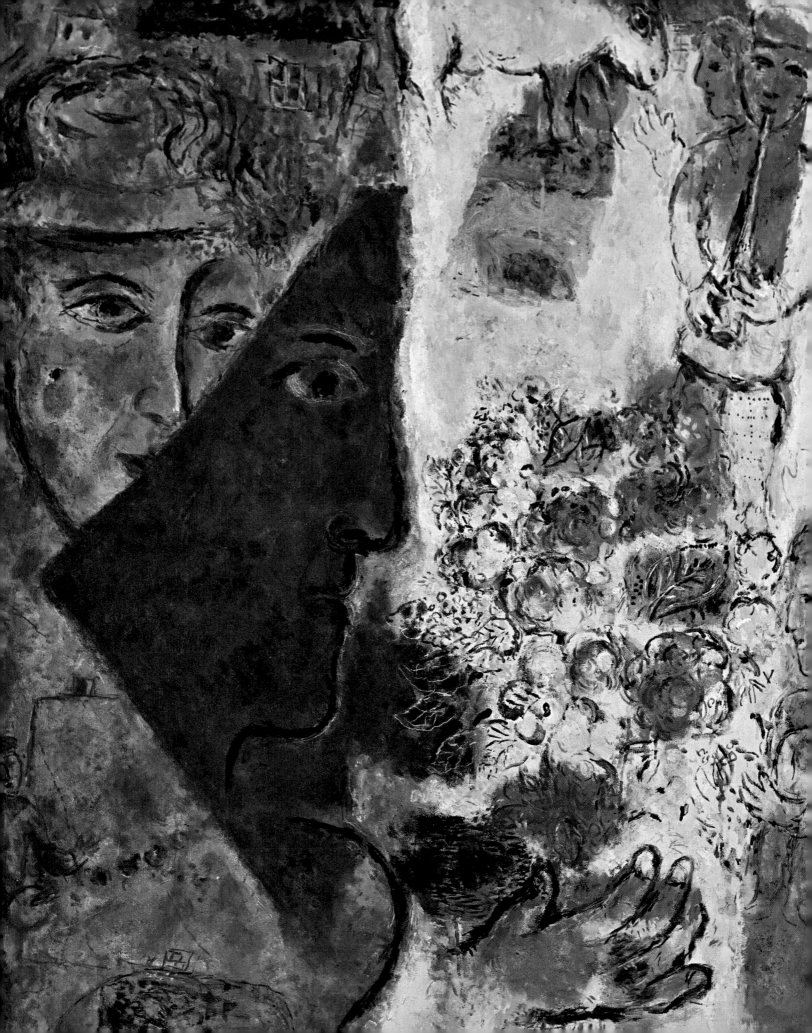

Chapter 9

Realms of Consciousness

Consciousness is a sea of shifting currents. From moment to moment it changes, rippling or churning, altering its drift as new sensations, ideas, emotions or memories surge into awareness. The thoughts flowing into a person's mind, the objects he sees and the sounds he hears, the feelings of pain or pleasure — all are interwoven into the endlessly fluctuating ocean that forms the conscious mind.

From the time man first pondered his universe, he has attempted to discover the source of this experience in the human body. Plato chose the head because the sphere, he claimed, was the perfect geometrical shape. Other ancient scholars proposed the heart, intestines, or liver as the wellspring of consciousness. Medieval man thought it arose from "animal spirit," a fluid supposedly made of air and nutrients from the liver, intestines and heart, and thought to be stored in the brain's ventricles. Seventeenth-century French philosopher René Descartes singled out the pineal gland, a teardrop of flesh in the back of the brain, as the seat of consciousness.

Philosophers and scientists agreed that consciousness was indeed connected with the brain. But how were they connected? Was consciousness entirely separate from the physical brain, or were they one and the same, merely different aspects of a single unit?

Today, scientists know that thoughts, feelings and sensations — the "stuff" of consciousness — are products of electrochemical activity in the brain. They have also discovered a basic and ancient mechanism in the depths of the brain that regulates the flow of consciousness.

Guardian of Consciousness

Stepping up to the service line, John McEnroe glances across court at Bjorn Borg. The world's two best male tennis players are at match point, deadlocked in their battle for the 1980 U.S. Open

From dreams' ethereal reaches Chagall's Blue Face *gazes to the warmth of simple earthly pleasures. The profuse interplay of feeling, dream, thought and memory colors the soaring tableau of consciousness.*

121

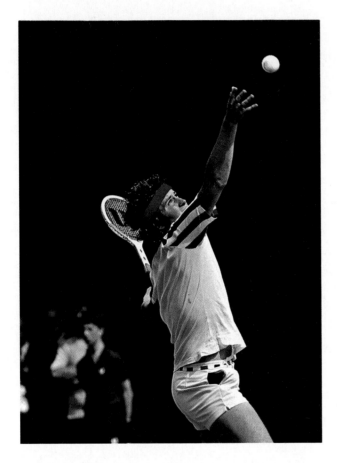

championship. As he prepares to serve, an intricate network of nerves in McEnroe's brain is busy whittling down his attention to a pinpoint, expelling from awareness a torrent of extraneous thoughts and sensations. Some of these surge from within the athlete's body: weary limbs begging for reprieve, thirst-proclaiming mouth glands, ruminations over a bad line call. From the external world pours information from his senses, telling of jeers from hostile onlookers, the slightly fuzzy feel of the tennis ball in his right hand, the muffled roar of a jet plane overhead. The nerve network screens from McEnroe's awareness all but a minute fraction of the messages clamoring for attention. At last, focused intently on ball and racquet, McEnroe rips a slashing serve across court in one fluid burst, waits for Borg's return, then strokes a stinging backhand smash far beyond Borg's reach, winning the point and match.

The web of nerves that creates the pinpoint concentration needed to win the U.S. Open championship operates continuously in all human beings during periods of alert wakefulness. It is a tangled, densely packed cluster of nerve cells known as the reticular formation. Roughly the size of the little finger, the reticular formation lies in the central core of the brainstem, that range of bulges which runs from the top of the spinal cord into the middle of the brain.

The reticular formation is, in essence, the physical basis of consciousness, the brain's chief watchguard. The cortex depends on impulses from the reticular formation for keeping us awake and alert. When stimulation of the reticular formation slackens, we sleep. Injury causes a coma, a prolonged state of unconsciousness.

Every second, 100 million messages bombard the brain carrying information from the body's senses. A few hundred, at most, are permitted through to brain regions above the brainstem. Of these, the conscious mind heeds a few. While a person may be partially aware of many sounds, smells or movements around him, concentration is limited to one sensation at a time. Without the reticular formation's alerting action, the cortex could not sort the significant messages from the trivial. The reticular formation continuously sifts and selects, forwarding only the essential, the unusual, the dangerous to the conscious mind.

Messages are sent as nerve impulses from sensory receptors in all parts of the body to the cortex through pathways that run up the spinal cord to the reticular formation. From there they are relayed to other brain regions. These pathways and the reticular formation are collectively called the reticular activating system — "RAS" for short. Most axons connecting nerve cells in the RAS are short, so that messages can be relayed quickly from one nerve cell to the next.

The reticular formation can both send and receive messages. If it suddenly spots one that merits attention, it shoots up an alert through ascending RAS pathways to receiving areas in the cortex. Timed to arrive simultaneously with the impulses sent directly from sensory receptors, the RAS alerts the cortex to these impulses. The cortex then identifies the specific message.

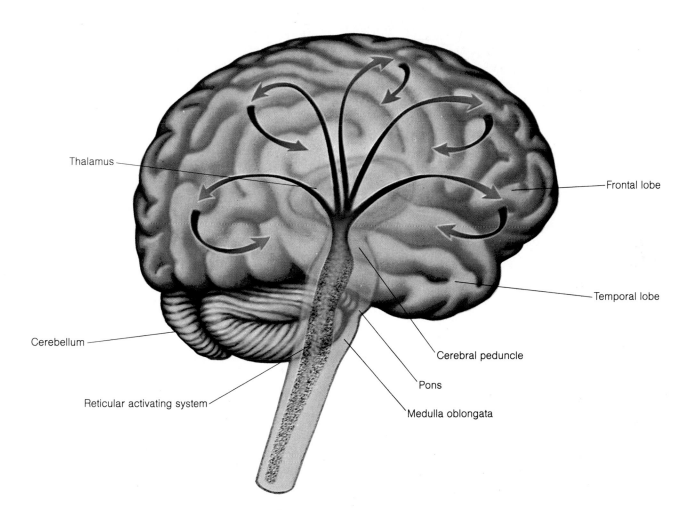

Thalamus

Frontal lobe

Cerebellum

Temporal lobe

Cerebral peduncle

Reticular activating system

Pons

Medulla oblongata

Gatekeeper to consciousness, spark of the mind, the reticular formation connects with major nerves in the spinal column and brain. It sorts the 100 million impulses that assault the brain each second, deflecting the trivial, letting the vital through to alert the mind. The mind cannot function without this catalytic bundle of cells. Damage to them results in coma — the loss of consciousness.

Circadian rhythms, the body's physiologic ebb and flow, hew to the earth's orbit. Traveling the solar day's 24-hour cycle, they drive the energies of every organism. Over a day, the powers of mind and body perpetually wax and wane in concert with shifts in light, temperature and place. Hence, most people naturally feel alert in the morning, drowsy at night, hungry at midday. Ninety-minute cycles, ultradian rhythms, spin through this larger pattern, sending subtler pulses of joy, awareness, hunger — and their opposites. Ultradian rhythms then ride on into night, through sleep cycles, too.

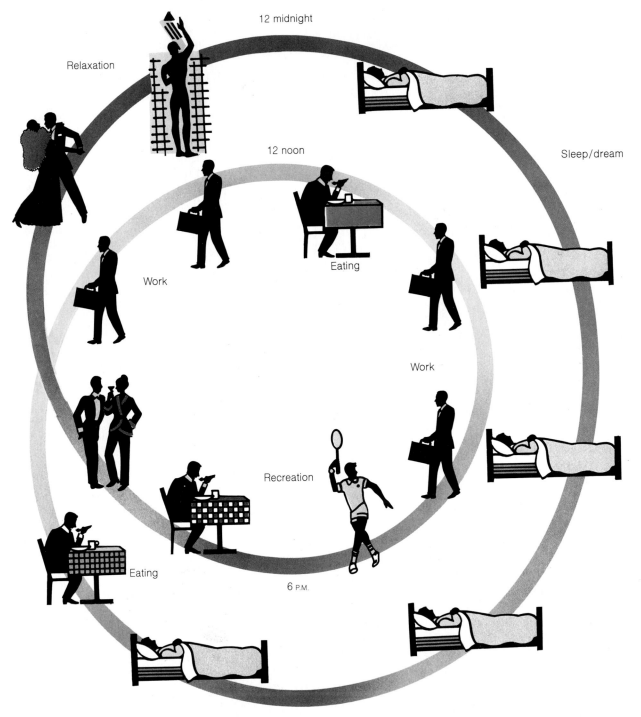

In its message-receiving capacity, the RAS obeys commands sent down from the cortex through descending RAS pathways. To enable John McEnroe to focus attention on his impending serve, the cortex commands the reticular formation to block out everything else. The RAS, in turn, passes the order to the spinal cord and the rest of his body. McEnroe's muscles become still, his mind clear and focused for the serve.

The RAS also regulates a process called habituation: The drilling of jackhammers assaulting a nearby street sets off an RAS alert, immediately capturing the brain's attention. But as soon as the sound's novelty has been recognized, the cortex directs the RAS to halt its alerting action.

The brain is stingy with its attention. Writes psychologist Charles Furst, "We can't afford to notice the way our socks feel on our feet." When an elevated train track running along Third Avenue in New York City was torn down, the city's police switchboard was flooded with calls. People who lived near the track complained of being awakened by an odd sensation. What actually woke them was the silence. Absence of the constant roar of passing trains forced them to "dishabituate" the noise.

Circadian Rhythms

In alternating rhythms of frenzy and relative calm, the brain's estimated ten billion nerve cells ignite, sending and receiving impulses at speeds ranging from 15 to 300 feet per second.

The rhythms that govern these interior stirrings affect all living organisms, and much of the physical world, too. Daily the sea tides rise and ebb. Every twenty-four hours, darkness extinguishes daylight. Summer's heat succumbs to the yearly chill of autumn. We grow hungry or tired, energetic or irritable, at fairly predictable intervals each day as the body's internal systems fluctuate. Body temperature usually peaks in the afternoon or evening, then drops to its lowest point between 2 A.M. and 5 A.M. Blood pressure, heartbeat, respiration, urine flow and levels of hormones and enzymes swing up and down rhythmically. In a healthy person, these body rhythms are well integrated. The flow of urine, for instance, normally plummets at night, allow-

ing the sleeper a long, uninterrupted rest. Sleep itself consists of various cycles.

These biological rhythms are regulated by a powerful internal clock, a circadian rhythm. Circadian is Latin for "around a day." Circadian rhythms are based roughly on the solar day, the shift of day into night as the earth revolves around the sun. Even when external indicators of time are absent, the body's clock keeps running. Actually, the body's cycle is closer to twenty-five hours. During experiments in sleep laboratories, subjects unaware of the time of day usually shift to a twenty-five-hour schedule, moving bedtimes and rising times forward one hour.

Circadian rhythms are so potent that their disruption can lead to irritability, depression or even physical illness. Jet lag, the result of high-speed travel across time zones, throws body rhythms out of kilter with the environment.

Some scientists believe people who suffer from depression are victims of out-of-phase body rhythms. The period of sleep in which dreaming takes place, called REM, often occurs prematurely in the sleep of depressed people.

Researchers now suspect that, due to the effects of circadian rhythms, exposure to a virus one day might cause mere fatigue, while exposure another day could result in illness. Similarly, certain drugs might be more potent when taken in the evening instead of earlier in the day.

The electrical activity of the brain seems to run in cycles of ninety minutes. During the day, periods of mental acuity alternate with intervals of listlessness or daydreaming, while at night dreaming and nondreaming sleep follow one another by turns. This cycle has also been detected in the patterns of hunger, epilepsy and increased mental disturbance among schizophrenics.

The brain's neuronal activity can be measured by an electroencephalograph, or EEG. The pattern recorded by the EEG is a "brainprint," unique to each individual. Throughout the day, this brainprint may change dozens of times as changes in states of consciousness alter the brain's pattern of electrical activity. Alertness, drowsiness, sleep, agitation or calm can be read from an EEG. Researchers also use the EEG to record the activity of the sleeping brain.

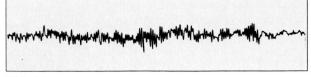

Wakefulness

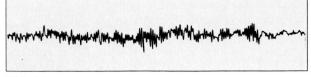

Stage 1

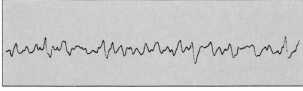

Stage 2

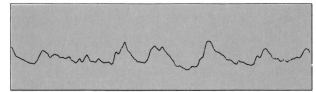

Stage 4

Changing brain waves trace the contours of sleep as it descends through NREM. The quick and steady alpha rhythm of wakeful relaxation (at top) yields to the erratic, low voltage pulses of Stage 1. High amplified bursts forming "sleep spindles" establish the tempo of Stage 2. The languorous, deep-troughed delta wave first appears in Stage 3, then dominates deep, Stage 4 sleep.

Thousands of overnight stays in sleep laboratories have created a portrait of sleep as a series of rhythms, each with its own brain-wave patterns. These rhythms fall into two major categories: REM and NREM (non-rem). NREM is a relatively peaceful slumber of varying depths, in which heartbeat, respiration and body temperature are slack and eye movements are slow and rolling. REM, or active sleep, is the time of irregular body activity, vivid dreaming and rapid eye movements, for which this sleep stage is named.

As a person drifts out of wakeful awareness, his muscles relax; heartbeat and breathing slacken. Random thoughts or images pass through his mind. The sleeper may feel he is floating. Perhaps he thinks he is still awake, but he is in the embrace of sleep's first stage. If his brain waves were recorded on an EEG, they would show the fast, low voltage pattern of Stage 1 sleep. The slightest noise could break this fragile slumber.

A few minutes later, the sleeper descends to Stage 2. Brain waves take on the appearance of wire spindles, tracing a dramatic design of peaks and valleys across the EEG paper. The eyes begin rolling slowly from side to side. Although Stage 2 sleep is deeper than Stage 1, it would still take only a slight noise to awaken someone.

Soon a few of the large, slow delta rhythms appear in the brain's wave pattern. This heralds the onset of Stage 3. The body becomes even more relaxed. Blood pressure, heart rate and body temperature decline. Only a loud noise would awaken the sleeper.

Roughly twenty minutes have elapsed since the onset of sleep. The fourth stage begins. Stage 4 is also called delta sleep because the slow, steady delta waves that first emerged in Stage 3 now dominate the brain-wave pattern. It would be extremely difficult to wake the sleeper from this deepest phase of sleep. Bed-wetting, sleeptalking and sleepwalking occur only in this stage.

Forty minutes have passed. For the next half hour or so, this sleep cycle will run backwards. From Stage 4, the sleeper drifts back into Stage 3, through Stage 2, then back to Stage 1. But this time, the brain's waves look more like the patterns of wakefulness. The first dream of the night is about to begin. The sleeper has entered

126

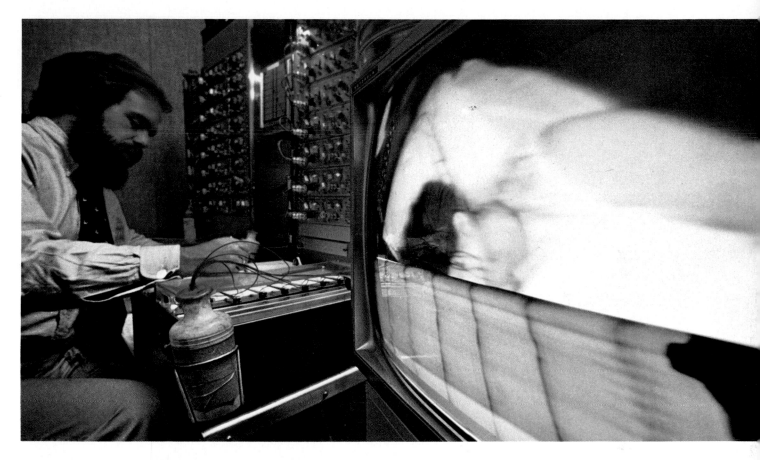

the REM period. In REM, the vital signs change suddenly and dramatically. Breathing, heartbeat and blood pressure become irregular. Under closed lids, the eyes dance back and forth as though the sleeper were watching a movie. In theory, this is exactly what happens during REM. According to the "scanning theory," the eyes move around as they follow the action of a dream. During REM, the brain sends a signal to the arms, legs and other large muscles to stop moving. This "sleep paralysis" prevents the body from acting out movements occurring in dreams.

The first REM period lasts nearly ten minutes. When it ends, the whole cycle repeats itself, usually four or five times each night. Each cycle lasts an average of ninety minutes. As the night wears on, REM periods lengthen, while NREM periods grow shorter. The final REM period of the night may last as long as one hour, or one-half to two-thirds of the total REM sleep each night.

Researchers have found great variation in human sleep requirements. While all people require sleep, some individuals are nonsomniacs, or "short" sleepers. Nonsomniacs are satisfied with one or two hours of sleep during a night.

Most adults average seven or eight hours each night. Infants, on the other hand, sleep nearly sixteen hours in scattered bursts throughout the day; most of this is REM sleep. By age five, children need ten or eleven hours. Adult sleep patterns become established during adolescence. Middle-aged people require slightly less sleep. At this time, too, deep sleep starts to decline. In old age, naps become frequent.

The need for sleep increases during pregnancy and illness. Anxiety, depression and physical or mental exertion also lengthen sleep. Researchers theorize that additional REM time — the result of longer sleep — restores the brain and helps it to integrate new experiences. In less stressful periods, demands on the brain are reduced, decreasing REM time. REM deprivation actually benefits some people. In a 1975 experiment at the Georgia Mental Health Institute, patients hospitalized for depression improved when they were deprived of REM sleep. Antidepressant drugs may be effective partly because they suppress REM sleep.

Some scientists believe personality accounts for basic differences in sleep requirements. One study found that long sleepers, those who sleep nine or more hours, are more anxious, introverted and less confident than short sleepers, who get six or less hours of sleep. Long sleepers, the researchers found, often use sleep as an escape from problems. Short sleepers are generally energetic, cheerful and self-confident, but are also less creative than long sleepers.

The Realm of Dream

Like the phenomenon of sleep itself, the function of dreams is unknown. Some scientists think the REM state in which vivid dreaming occurs plays a vital role in keeping the central nervous system in good working order. Others view dreams primarily as a means for solving conflicts. Newer theories assign dreams the role of synthesizing memories and new information.

Theories about the meaning of dreams are as abundant as speculation about their ultimate function. People in many modern societies share the view of the ancient Greeks and Hebrews that dreams are portents of the future. Some tribal societies regard the dream world as another plane of reality, equal to the waking world. They believe a person who commits an illegal or immoral act in a dream deserves punishment for it.

Of all theories about the meaning of dreams, perhaps none has influenced modern attitudes more than the one formulated by Sigmund Freud, the father of psychoanalysis. Freud believed that in dreams, the primitive urges we repress during the day are transformed into disguised symbols. According to Freud, the wishes these symbols represent are too repugnant for the conscious mind. Freud assigned fixed symbolic meanings, mostly sexual in nature, to many dream objects, interpreting long objects as phallic symbols, and hollow forms as female symbols.

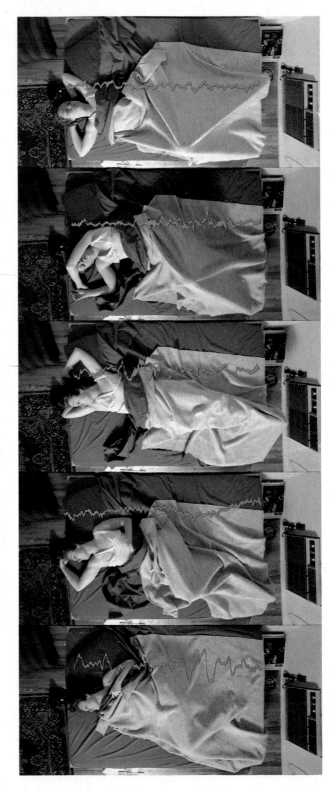

Rising to touch the dawn, sleep cycles grow less deep as night unfolds. REM periods, meanwhile, lengthen and intensify, painting as much as an hour of the final 90-minute cycle with vivid dreams.

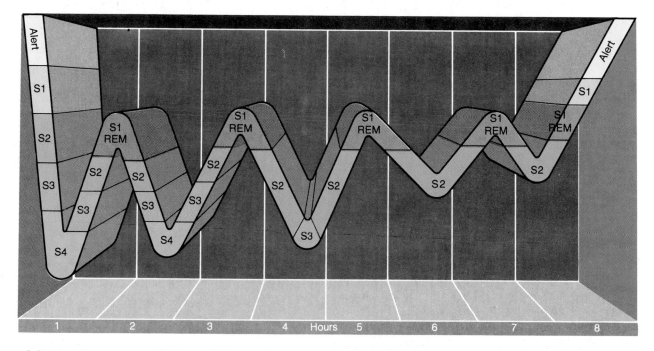

Many scientists now believe dreaming is more a physiological process than a psychological one. According to the "activation-synthesis" theory, dreams are the brain's attempt to impose meaning on the bewildering array of electrical impulses that shoot up to the cortex from the lower brain during REM periods. This theory, proposed by J. Allan Hobson and Robert McCarley of the Neurophysiology Laboratory, Massachusetts Mental Health Center, is based on findings that suggest sleep is controlled by the pons, a clump of nerve fibers in the midbrain. At the onset of REM, the giant cells of the pons begin firing. Excitation rapidly spreads to nearby cells and then to the cerebral cortex. Drawing on its inventory of memories, the cortex assembles these nerve impulses into a sensible pattern, creating what the sleeper experiences as a dream.

Many of the bizarre qualities of dreams may be understood as the struggle of the cortex to yoke together the disparate signals it receives from neuron firings in the lower brain. An instantaneous trip from the backyard to Peking, or the sudden transformation of a dream character from human to animal occurs when one sequence of nerve-cell firings ends and another begins. Hobson and McCarley do not dismiss dreams as

strictly physiological events. The way in which the brain assembles and interprets the flurry of neuronal impulses, they believe, is unique to each individual, the product of one's personality, emotions and experiences.

Under ordinary circumstances dreams occur at least once during every REM period. Sleep lasting seven or eight hours can produce a dozen or more dreams. Only one person in three, however, recalls any dream. Studies suggest personality plays a decisive role in the ability to remember dreams. Introspective people have better dream recall than those who are less attentive to their feelings. Waking conditions also affect the recall of dreams. Waking from a REM period increases the likelihood of remembering a dream. Dream recall is probably higher on weekends when there is more time to linger in bed.

Reports from thousands of sleep subjects awakened from all stages of sleep show that dreams occur not only in REM periods but in other sleep stages as well. REM dreams, however, are much more vivid and detailed.

Most people, places and objects in dreams are familiar to the dreamer. Everyday activities and events are more common than exotic ones. Dreams often include experiences that occurred

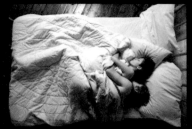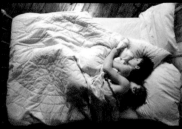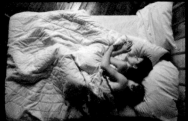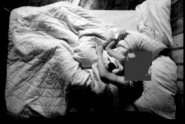
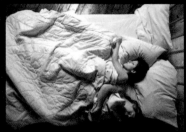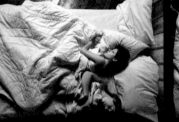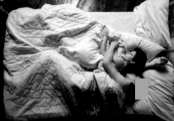
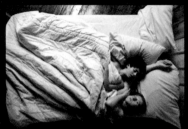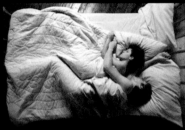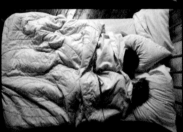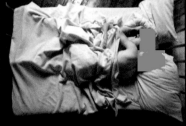
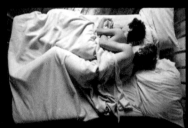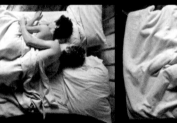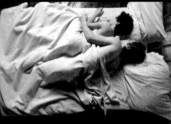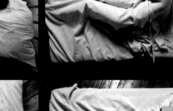
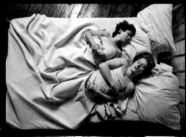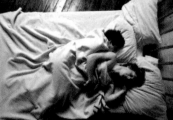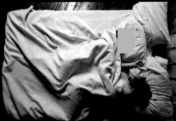
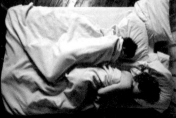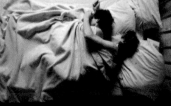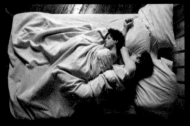
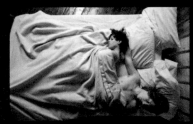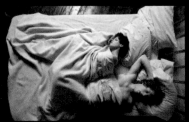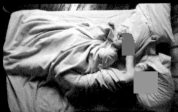

on the preceding day. Surprisingly, however, trivial events seem to have greater influence on dream content than do more significant ones, especially in the night's early dreams. Toward morning, dreams become less prosaic, drawing from the brain's store of childhood memories.

Some scientists think dreams are primarily the product of the right hemisphere of the brain, the side that controls nonverbal, spatial and emotional functions. It is more active than the left during REM. People with right-hemisphere damage also have reported loss of vivid dreaming.

Boundaries of Consciousness

Because dreaming is a regular nightly occurrence, it falls within the realms of consciousness one would consider ordinary. But the bizarre qualities of dreams — distortions of time, space and events — evoke less common states of awareness, where perceptions and fantasies are merged, the extraordinary becomes commonplace and eerie illusions imitate reality. From the beginning of time, mankind has sought such transcendence from ordinary consciousness.

The desire to experience other states of consciousness is probably innate, according to psychologist Andrew Weil. In *The Natural Mind* Weil writes: "Anyone who watches very young children . . . will find them regularly practicing techniques that induce striking changes in mental states. Three- and four-year-olds . . . commonly whirl themselves into . . . stupors. They hyperventilate and have other children squeeze them around the chest until they faint."

While some altered states have physiological correlates — distinctive brain waves or changes in vital signs — others have no observable bodily effects. Too, what feels like an altered state to one person can seem very ordinary to another. The daydreamer's detachment from his surroundings is similar to many altered states, yet some people consider daydreaming a normal part of their waking consciousness. Psychologist Charles Tart defines an altered state as a "qualitative alteration in the overall pattern of mental functioning . . . that the experiencer feels."

Since the 1960s, many people have experimented with chemicals, taking psychoactive or

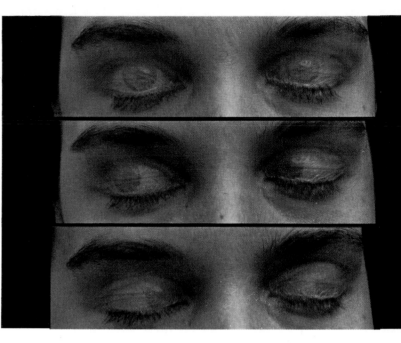

Rapid eye movement, REM, only occurs during dreams. Discovered less than 30 years ago, REM still puzzles researchers. Some think it an outward sign of this sleep stage's enhanced brain activity. Others believe it an effort by the sleeper to scan the dream's action.

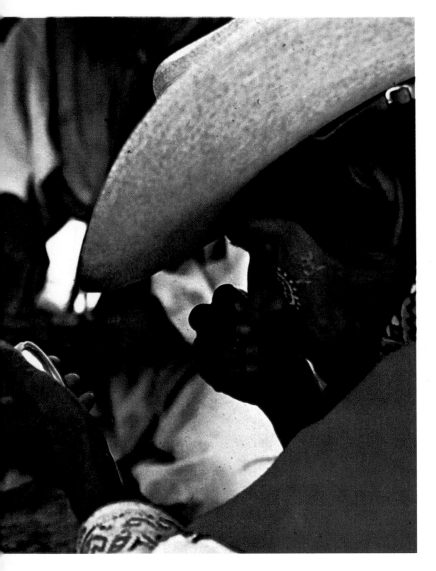

*"We take peyote to find our lives,"
say Mexico's Huichol Indians.
Above, a Huichol paints his face as
part of a religious rite, copying a
drug-inspired vision. Its chemical
interactions constant, the brain
unfailingly sees similar geometric
patterns while in the velvety grasp
of a drug like peyote. These
recurrent images are called
hallucinogenic form constants.*

perception-distorting drugs. Because lysergic acid diethylamide (LSD), marijuana, amphetamines and other mind-altering drugs can generate symptoms of psychoses along with expansion of consciousness, their effects are unpredictable.

Many respected twentieth-century figures have taken mind-altering drugs. In *The Doors of Perception*, Aldous Huxley described a revelation he had while under the influence of mescaline, a powerful hallucinogen similar in effect to LSD. While staring at a flower arrangement, he "was not looking now at an unusual flower arrangement. I was seeing what Adam had seen on the morning of his creation — the miracle, moment by moment, of naked existence."

William James, the American philosopher and psychologist, and Sigmund Freud also experimented with psychoactive drugs. James described his experience with nitrous oxide, an anesthetic known as laughing gas, as "intense metaphysical illumination." Freud wrote of the "exhilaration" and "lasting euphoria" of cocaine. But sufficient quantities of amphetamines and cocaine can produce terrifying hallucinations. Although he praised cocaine's euphoria, Freud also hallucinated "bugs . . . small animals moving in the skin."

Scientists believe many psychoactive drugs interfere with the electrochemical transmissions between the brain's neurons. The neurons become artificially overstimulated, disrupting the normal rhythm of nerve impulses from cell to cell. The result is distorted perception of time, space and matter.

Some of the effects of psychoactive drugs resemble symptoms of acute schizophrenia. The paranoia, hallucinations and loss of identity in both the drug experience and schizophrenia suggest to some researchers that certain psychoactive drugs, such as amphetamines, could be the chemical key to schizophrenia. Other scientists note differences between drug-induced madness and symptoms of schizophrenia. The broken thought processes of schizophrenia are generally absent from the drug experience. Drug hallucinations, too, are usually visual, while most schizophrenic hallucinations are auditory.

Unusual physical or emotional stress — extreme hunger or thirst, lack of sleep, severe pain,

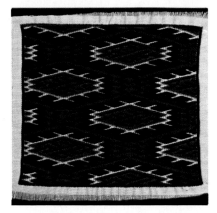

A sampling of form constants embroidered by peyote appears in Huichol textiles.

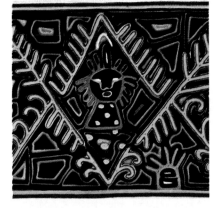

These include, from top to bottom: lattice, spiral, tunnel and cobweb.

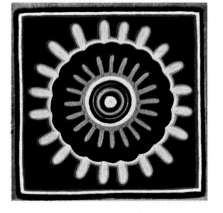

Hallucinogens spawn like geometric patterns universally, but detail varies between cultures.

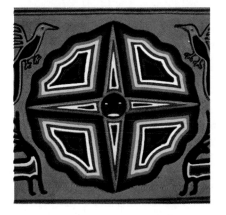

While the Huichol see animals, the Dutch, for example, might see tulips.

fever or sensory deprivation — can also trigger hallucinations. The monotony of driving can cause truck drivers to hallucinate spiders on their windshields and airplane pilots to "see" turbulence in calm skies.

An early researcher of hallucinations, Heinrich Kluver, found that people using mescaline consistently described the forms of visual hallucinations as four basic shapes — lattice, spiral, cobweb or tunnel. Later, he and other investigators discovered that those who suffered epilepsy, psychotic episodes, dizziness or migraine headaches experienced the same visual hallucinations. Mexico's Huichol Indians, who ritually take peyote, use these same forms in their art.

According to psychiatrist L. Jolyon West of the University of California at Los Angeles, hallucinations are memory traces that are released into awareness when the level or variety of sensory information sent to the brain drops below a certain point. Normally, West theorizes, the brain's memory stores are held in check by adequate sensory stimulation. Other scientists think hallucinations are associated with excitation of the central nervous system along with a malfunction of the reticular formation.

Altered states of consciousness can also be achieved through various techniques of meditation. All methods share certain features: In quiet surroundings, the meditator concentrates on a single point of focus — a word, shape, idea, question or, perhaps, his own breathing. Such narrowed attention compels the mind to shift from its customary busy state to one of passive receptiveness. As the mind's activity is stilled, the meditator becomes detached from thought. Some practitioners seek relaxation and a sense of well-being. Others, particularly those who practice a religion in which meditation plays a central role, aspire to mystical states.

Scientific findings on meditation are contradictory. In one study, subjects showed reductions in blood pressure, heart rate and oxygen consumption, intensified alpha brain waves and other signs of deep relaxation. The meditators seemed to produce a unique consciousness, a state of deep, though wakeful, relaxation. This "relaxation response," the scientists theorized, is the

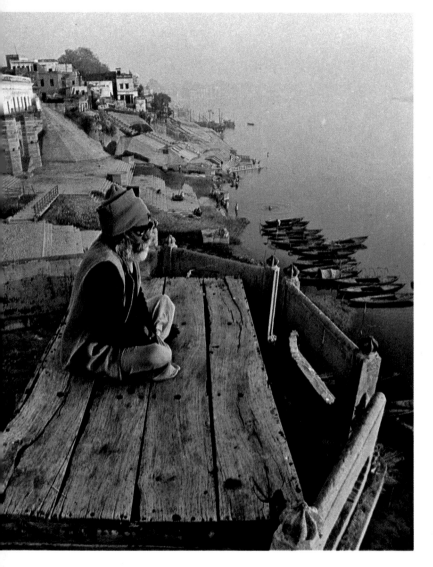

Deep in meditation, a yogi sits high over India's Ganges River. The practice, in slowing such functions as heart rate and oxygen use, steels the mind. Some master yogis can lie peaceably on a bed of nails.

reverse of the fight-or-flight reaction that causes blood pressure, heart rate and oxygen consumption to soar during stress. Other investigators dispute that meditation is a unique state.

There is little question, however, that meditation can affect bodily functions, often in dramatic ways. Yogis train themselves to enter states in which the sensation of pain is somehow blocked. They are then able to submerge their hands in extremely cold water or lie on beds of nails without experiencing discomfort.

Similar feats of mind over body have been credited to the hypnotic trance. Hypnotic suggestions can bring about changes in heart rate, stop bleeding, increase muscular strength, or lower one's sensitivity to pain. Hypnosis has cured phobias and caused warts to disappear spontaneously. Researchers suggest hypnosis allows subjects to become aware of submerged memories and somehow enables them to gain control over heartbeat, breathing, digestion and glandular activity — involuntary processes not normally subject to conscious control. Although the term hypnosis is taken from the Greek *hypnos*, for "sleep," it bears little resemblance to sleep states. Rather, like meditation, it couples physical relaxation with mental concentration.

Hypnosis has been used as an anesthetic during surgery, as a psychoanalytic device to delve into the unconscious and as a means for treating shell-shocked soldiers. Medical and psychiatric associations have approved its practice, and dental and medical schools now teach it. Many police departments employ hypnotists to prod the memories of crime witnesses.

But beneath the current ardor for hypnosis lies a dense layer of skepticism. Feats achieved through hypnosis have been duplicated by unhypnotized subjects who are motivated and given the appropriate suggestions. Psychologist Theodore Barber, a prominent skeptic, states: "Since no test has been able to demonstrate the existence of the hypnotic state, there is no reason to assume that there *is* such a state."

A newer and equally controversial technique for consciously regulating physical processes is biofeedback. Sophisticated electronic equipment monitors a person's brain waves, blood pressure and other involuntary activities, displaying information, or feedback, about them with flashing lights, meter needles and audio devices. The biofeedback subject learns to control these activities through passive concentration, a relaxed mental state allowing the mind to respond to the audio-visual display and modify the particular physical process. It seems relaxation, rather than conscious effort, is the key to successful biofeedback. To encourage relaxation, biofeedback subjects are instructed to visualize soothing activities such as sun-bathing on a deserted beach or walking through a field of flowers.

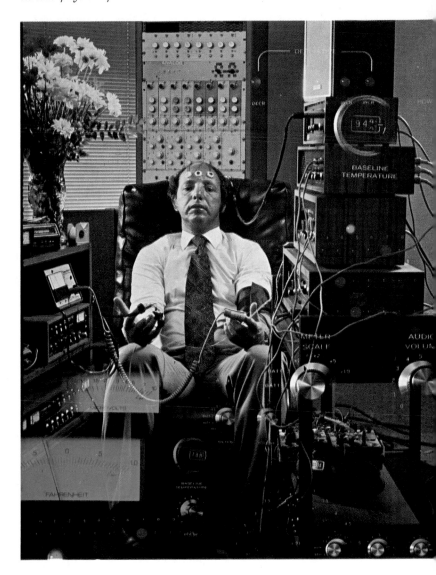

Biofeedback's most successful medical applications have been in the area of muscle control. With the aid of an electromyograph (EMG), a device that measures muscle tension, biofeedback subjects can control healthy muscles and, in some cases, regain the use of diseased ones. Victims of neuromuscular disorders such as palsy and stroke-induced paralysis also benefit from biofeedback by learning to use alternate neural passages to control the movement of their limbs.

Other medical applications of biofeedback include the treatment of epilepsy and migraine headaches. Some epileptics have dramatically reduced the number of seizures by learning to modify the brain's electrical activity. Those suffering from migraine headaches, caused by expansion of the blood vessels around the brain, have obtained relief by learning to raise the temperature of their hands. This restores balance to the circulatory system by increasing the flow of blood to the hands and decreasing the amount of blood in the vessels that supply the brain.

Critics of biofeedback note that learning often stops after training is completed. Too, while biofeedback might be useful in reducing high blood pressure, they point out, it does not cure hypertension. But many scientists agree with physiologist Barbara Brown: "It seems likely that in the future we will be able to control many of the numerous specific brain waves as well as patterns of brain waves that reflect the activities of our minds and states of consciousness. We should be able to become so aware of the best states of mind and body that we can achieve both internal harmony and harmony with the universe."

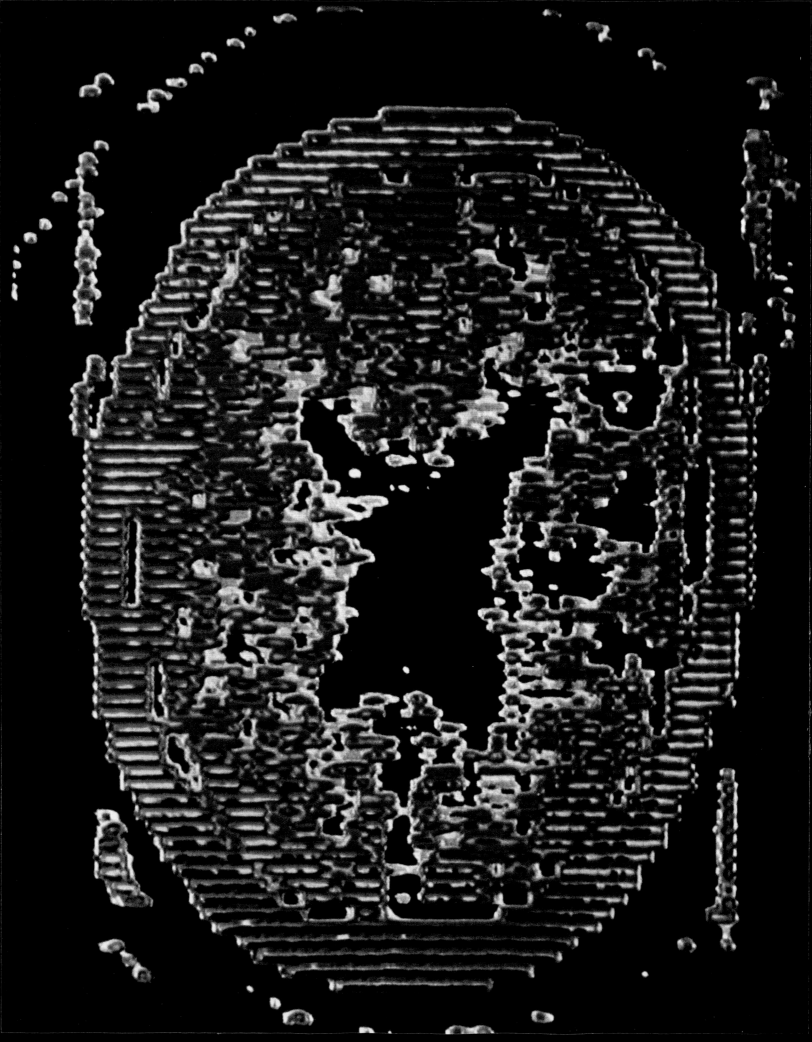

Chapter 10

The Unfolding Tapestry

In convoluted folds inside man's head lies the most complex living substance known. Buried within the winding, pink gray coils of the human brain is the essence of life itself. What Plato called the "divinest part of us" is also the most mysterious. Worldly-wise, capable of devising the technology for sending rockets into space or splitting atoms, the brain is at the same time amazingly ignorant of its own workings.

But in research, diagnosis and treatment, the neurosciences are advancing with unprecedented speed. Today, the methods of diagnosing and treating brain disorders employ highly sophisticated computers, mammoth particle accelerators, microminiaturized surgical tools and X-ray scanners capable of producing thousands of anatomical cross sections per second. Modern medicine seeks to invent better techniques for viewing the brain's interior without actually entering it.

The development of the CAT scanner has revolutionized the diagnosis of brain disorders. With CAT, or computerized axial tomography, doctors can see into the deepest recesses of their patients' brains. The scanner's high-speed computer projects a sharply focused, highly detailed tomogram, or cross section, of the patient's brain onto a television screen. The picture allows the doctor to diagnose quickly and accurately a suspected tumor, blood clot or hemorrhage. The scanner also detects birth defects, brain damage characteristic of certain forms of senility and distinguishes between old and new strokes.

Before the advent of the brain scanner in the early 1970s, many brain disorders were difficult or impossible to detect by conventional X-ray techniques. Conventional X-rays do not reveal depth, making it difficult to distinguish between the overlapping structures of the brain's soft tissues. In trying to diagnose a tumor, X-rays were taken from many different angles. Even then, a tumor might not show up because it has nearly

The brain in geometric brilliance emerges from an X-ray composite called CAT. Introduced in 1973, CAT paints brain tissue varying hues based on relative density. This yields intricate internal detail, which enhances the hunt for such intruders as infection and tumors.

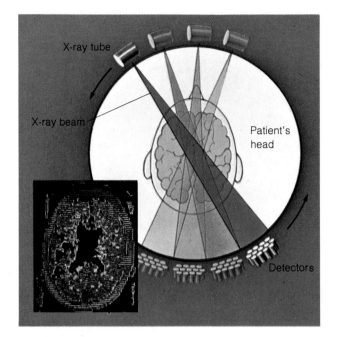

By mathematically analyzing the difference between the total radiation emitted and the amount hitting the detectors, the computer reconstructs what happens to the beams — where and how much they are absorbed — as they pass through the brain. And, like slicing an onion and turning the pieces to see the concentric pattern inside, the scanner's computer rotates the mathematical information ninety degrees. The picture it projects onto the screen is a view of the brain as if one were looking through it and seeing the broad side of a single slice. A series of scans allows the doctor to peer into layer after layer of his patient's brain. Additional scans taken from other angles can be used to pinpoint extremely small abnormalities of brain tissue.

Beyond CAT

But CAT's dazzle will soon be competing with a machine just making its debut. The most complex and versatile medical instrument ever invented, the Dynamic Spatial Reconstructor, or DSR, is a highly sophisticated X-ray machine. Like CAT, DSR uses a computer to assemble X-ray pictures of the body into composite video images. While CAT shows slices, DSR presents a three-dimensional anatomical panorama, the end product of an elaborate electronic procedure that mathematically dices and reassembles the body.

Like an electronic knife, DSR can pictorially slice open an organ and expose its interior, allowing doctors to watch it in motion, pulsing with the flow of blood and oxygen. To study the brain, doctors can cut it open, turn it on its side or upside down, and enlarge the image. DSR also offers doctors a choice of stop-action, replay, high-speed or slow-motion viewing. During a DSR scan, twenty-eight X-ray guns revolve around the patient, each firing sixty times per second. In five seconds, DSR can produce 75,000 cross sections, while CAT, in that time, can only make one. A scan that would take CAT several minutes can be completed by DSR in seconds.

DSR's speed enables doctors to study body functions, not just structure. They can follow the flow of blood through the brain, detecting early signs of a stroke and other disorders. Scientists have just begun experimental DSR scans of peo-

Like earth around sun, CAT circles the head, taking myriad images. The result, a cross section of the brain, defines each part of the organ. Common X-rays can only blur them into black and white masses.

the same density as the healthy tissue in which it is imbedded. The CAT scanner not only finds and determines the size of the tumor, but a series of scans can distinguish a spreading from a non-spreading tumor. As it scans, the machine computes the densities of different brain tissues.

Despite the variety of CAT scanners in use today, all work in the same basic way. Placed on a table in front of the doughnut-shaped scanner, the patient is positioned so that his head projects through the hole. Above his head, an X-ray tube rotates along a circular path. The rotating scanner sweeps specific amounts of X-ray beams along a pencil-thin line through the head. As the beams pass through the head, the brain's soft tissues absorb small amounts of radiation, depending on the density of the tissue. Once the beams pass through the brain, they are converted by light-sensitive crystal detectors to electronic signals that are transmitted to the scanner's computer.

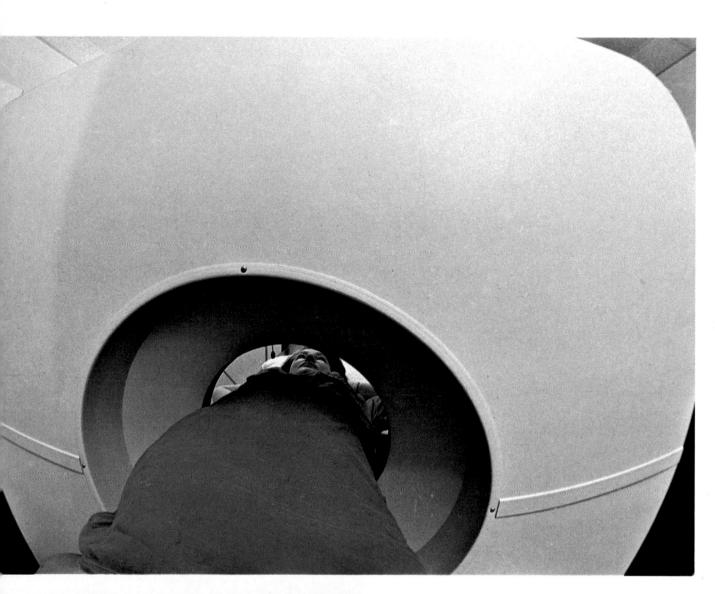

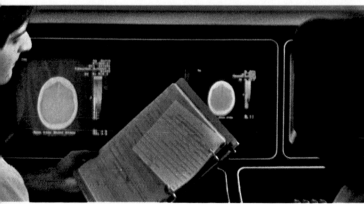

In CAT's iron halo, a patient undergoes a scan. The procedure, often lasting a half-hour, reads out on monitors, at left. CAT accounts for a sizable portion of U.S. health care costs, leading some to suspect its indiscriminate use. Proponents see the machines as revolutionary tools which reduce hospital stays and reliance on riskier diagnostic tests.

PETT receptors, below, register the gamma rays produced as brain tissue absorbs isotope. PETT scans, at right, show, left to right, oxygen use, blood volume and blood flow to aid doctors in diagnosis.

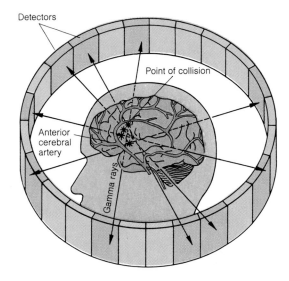

Detectors

Point of collision

Anterior cerebral artery

Gamma rays

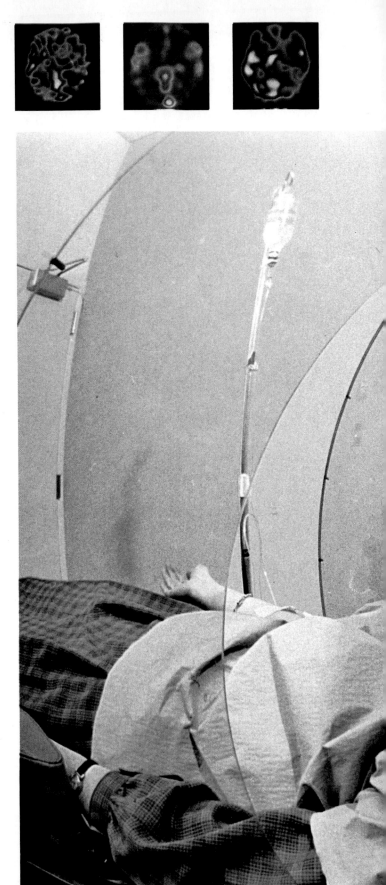

ple at the Mayo Clinic in Rochester, Minnesota, where the machine was developed. The cost of this agile instrument, $3 to 5 million, could prove a drawback to its ever becoming a standard diagnostic tool for hospitals.

CAT, DSR and other X-ray techniques use radiation — the emission of particles or waves from certain elements — to take pictures of body tissue. Medicine also employs radiation in another diagnostic test, the radioisotope scan. Radioisotope scanning charts the body's chemical activity. Isotopes are chemical elements with nearly identical chemical properties but different atomic weights. Isotopes which are not stable are radioactive; they disintegrate, emitting radiation. Doctors trace the course of the injected radioisotope through the body. Unusually large or small concentrations in specific areas can indicate disease. Like DSR, radioisotope scans can provide early warning of disease.

Although radioisotope scans have been used diagnostically since the 1950s, their value was limited by poor image quality. New computer imaging techniques similar to those used in CAT have made possible a sophisticated version of radioisotope scanning called PETT, or positron-emission transaxial tomography.

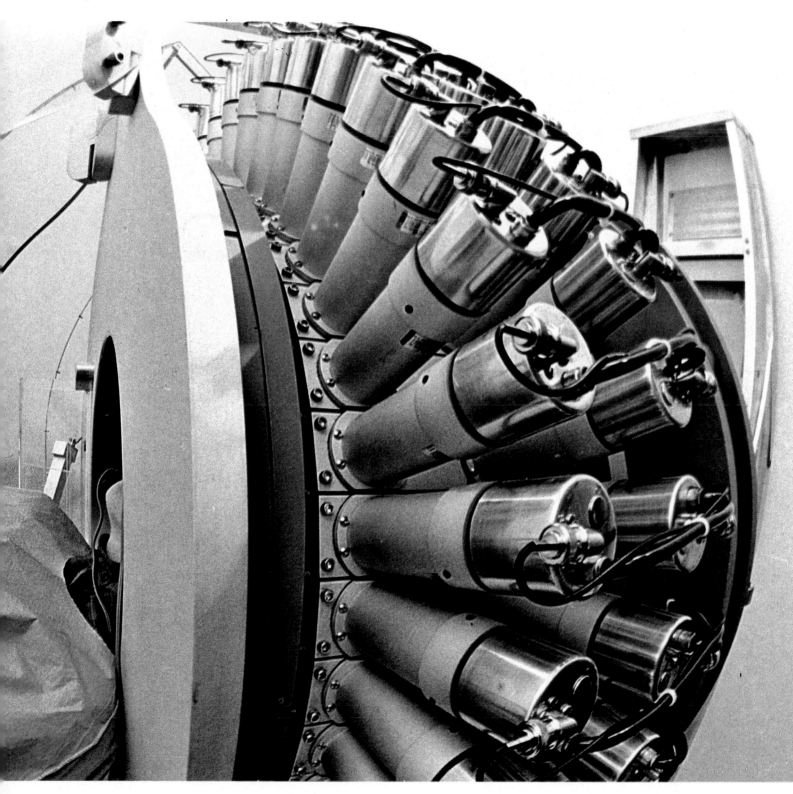

A patient's head disappears into the maw of a PETT scanner bristling with photon detectors. Each machine costs several million dollars and requires thirty people to produce one diagnostic scan.

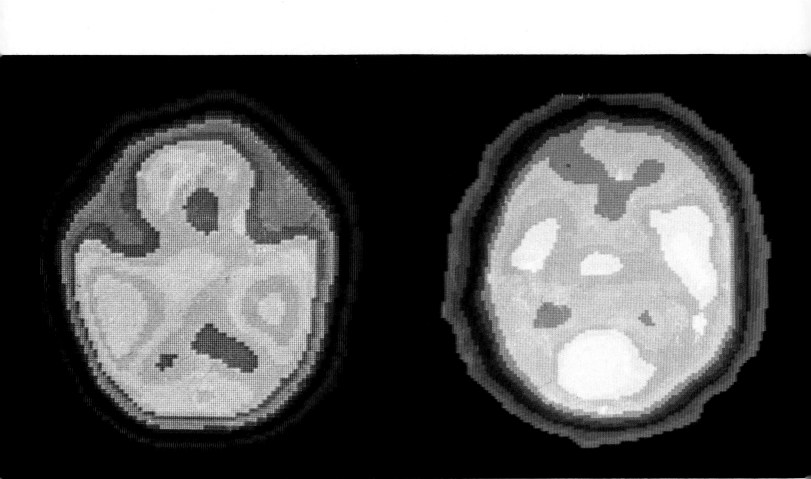

Masks of illness lift under the scrutiny of PETT. Symmetrical shapes and colors signal normal behavior at left, while orange shape in frontal lobe at top of middle scan shows schizophrenia. At right, as manic depression consumes much glucose, white areas eat toward the brain's center. Doctors see PETT as a great technological hope for pinpointing both mental illness and its prescriptive remedy.

An injected radioactive isotope moving through the body emits positive electrons, or positrons, which collide with negatively charged electrons in body cells. As the particles annihilate each other, they release gamma rays in opposite directions. After detecting and recording them, a computer then turns the information into a colored biochemical map of the body's metabolism, the conversion of substances into energy.

Still experimental, PETT scanning may not become a clinical tool for several years. But it has already provided information about the body never before available. Using PETT, doctors can study the effects of drugs within specific body organs, identify brain areas damaged by stroke or concussion and determine which brain regions are agitated during epileptic seizures.

Early PETT tests have shed light on the physiology of mental illness. In tests conducted at Brookhaven National Laboratory on Long Island,

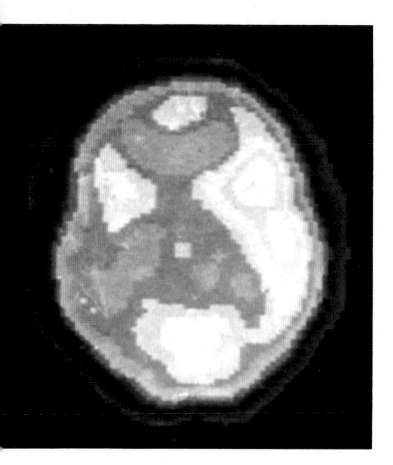

Another new diagnostic brain tool, nuclear magnetic resonance (NMR), has for decades been one of the chemist's chief methods for analyzing the composition of unknown substances. To study the body's hydrogen density, NMR uses hydrogen atoms in a magnetic field. These atoms emit electrical signals when a beam of high energy is applied to the field. The signals, processed by computer, are converted into a picture of the biochemistry of brain and body.

Until the early 1970s, NMR instruments could measure objects no longer than a quarter of an inch. But the recent enlargement of NMR equipment has made possible the scanning of the whole human body.

Measuring the electrical activity of the brain is another way of finding disorders and exploring brain function. Evoked potentials, minute changes in electrical voltage, are the brain's response to sensory stimuli. At one-tenth the amplitude of normal brain waves — a mere zephyr in the mental hurricane — an evoked potential must be winnowed out from the brain's electrical activity like a radio signal from an ocean of static. To identify an evoked potential, a computer averages a person's brain waves while he is repeatedly presented with a particular stimulus — a flash of light, identifiable shapes or a series of clicking noises. After hundreds of presentations, the computer can then identify the specific brain waves created by the stimulus.

Because evoked-potentials testing is quick and requires no verbal response, it is ideal for detecting vision and hearing defects in newborn infants. Early diagnosis of such abnormalities can prevent life-long impairment.

Scientists have found, through these studies, that the mental processes of attention, expectancy and split-second decision making each create different brain waves. They have even identified a specific signal that occurs only when a person has been confronted with nonsense.

Evoked potentials are now used to determine the cause of a child's poor scholastic performance. Biologically based learning disorders produce abnormal brain waves. Doctors also use evoked potentials to assess brain damage from stroke and injury, to diagnose brain tumors and

New York, schizophrenic and manic-depressive patients were injected with a radioactive substance similar to glucose, the brain's chief source of fuel. PETT, scanning cross sections of the brain, revealed areas of high, low or normal glucose consumption. The PETT scans of the schizophrenic patients showed decreased activity in certain brain areas, while the manic-depressive patients experienced increased brain activity during manic phases.

The PETT scan could eventually become a routine part of psychiatric diagnosis, proving valuable in diagnosing patients who show symptoms of more than one kind of mental illness.

Scientists are also using PETT scans to explore the healthy brain. By detecting and recording changes in glucose consumption within the brain, PETT is helping scientists to identify specific areas which are involved in both sensory and motor activities.

multiple sclerosis and to predict if and when a comatose patient will regain consciousness.

In their quest to understand how nerve pathways in the brain work, some scientists have embarked on a meticulous, painstaking journey through individual brain cells. Implanting fine-tipped microelectrodes into single neurons, these researchers record each cell's reaction to a specific sensory stimulus. Used to study animal brain functions, single-cell microelectrode recording gives scientists a better understanding of vision.

Pathways of Sight

Using microelectrode recordings, Harvard psychologists David Hubel and Torsten Wiesel have drawn a map of the primary visual cortex, the region at the back of the cerebrum where signals from the retina are interpreted. Step by step, they have traced the neural pathways of sight, finding an intricate arrangement of brain cells. Many cells, they discovered, have specialized functions, firing only in response to light presented at a certain angle, while others respond to particular shades of color or specific directions of movement. Hubel and Wiesel also found that some cells receive signals mostly from one eye, while others respond equally to both. Cells are grouped in "ocular dominance columns" according to which eye they respond to best.

Vision is not the only brain process which has been illuminated by microelectrode experiments. Two Russian scientists discovered the cellular basis for the phenomenon called habituation. The sound of a lawn mower is noticed for the first few moments after it begins, but then fades out of conscious awareness as the listener becomes habituated to it. The scientists found specific "novelty-recording" cells which fire only in response to a novel stimulus. Once the stimulus has been repeated, these cells stop firing.

Important progress in the treatment of brain disorders has also been achieved through drug research. L-dopa, a drug which raises dopamine levels in the brain, has been used since the 1960s to relieve the muscular tremors and rigidity of Parkinson's disease (a condition linked to a deficiency of the brain chemical, dopamine). But the negative side effects of the drug impelled re-

searchers to find a better treatment. They have now discovered ways to combine L-dopa with a counteracting drug, enabling doctors to fit the formula to the needs of an individual patient.

The recent development of ara-A, a drug used to combat the deadly brain virus herpes encephalitis marks a medical milestone. Virtually all other antiviral drugs harm body cells. In 1977, scientists reported that ara-A reduced deaths and neurological damage from herpes encephalitis without apparent cell damage.

Researchers are also seeking a cure for multiple sclerosis (MS), a disease which gradually destroys the fatlike myelin sheath surrounding nerve fibers. Some scientists believe the disease arises when a person becomes immune, for unknown reasons, to a brain protein called myelin basic protein. But they found this same substance, when put in salt solution, desensitized the immune cells of animals with an MS-like disease and cured them. In a study in progress at the University of Toronto, MS patients admitted to the hospital during acute attacks are injected with myelin basic protein extracted from the nervous systems of cattle. Dr. E. H. Eylar, the scientist conducting the study, describes preliminary results as encouraging, especially for patients treated in early stages of the disease.

Spinal cord injuries might someday be alleviated by naloxone, a drug commonly used to reverse the effects of opiates. Although useless for those already paralyzed, the drug appears to prevent or decrease paralysis when given to animals in shock following a spinal cord injury. Researchers suspect naloxone prevents paralysis by restoring normal blood pressure after shock, which in turn stimulates the flow of blood to the spinal cord.

Mending Minute Blood Vessels

Advances in neurosurgical techniques have kept stride with drug research. Microsurgery is saving the lives of many potential victims of stroke, the most common brain injury. Combining modern improvements in microscope optics with precision microinstruments, surgeons are now able to restore circulation to obstructed areas of the brain. Within the brain a multitude of tiny arteries supplies life-giving oxygen. If enough blood

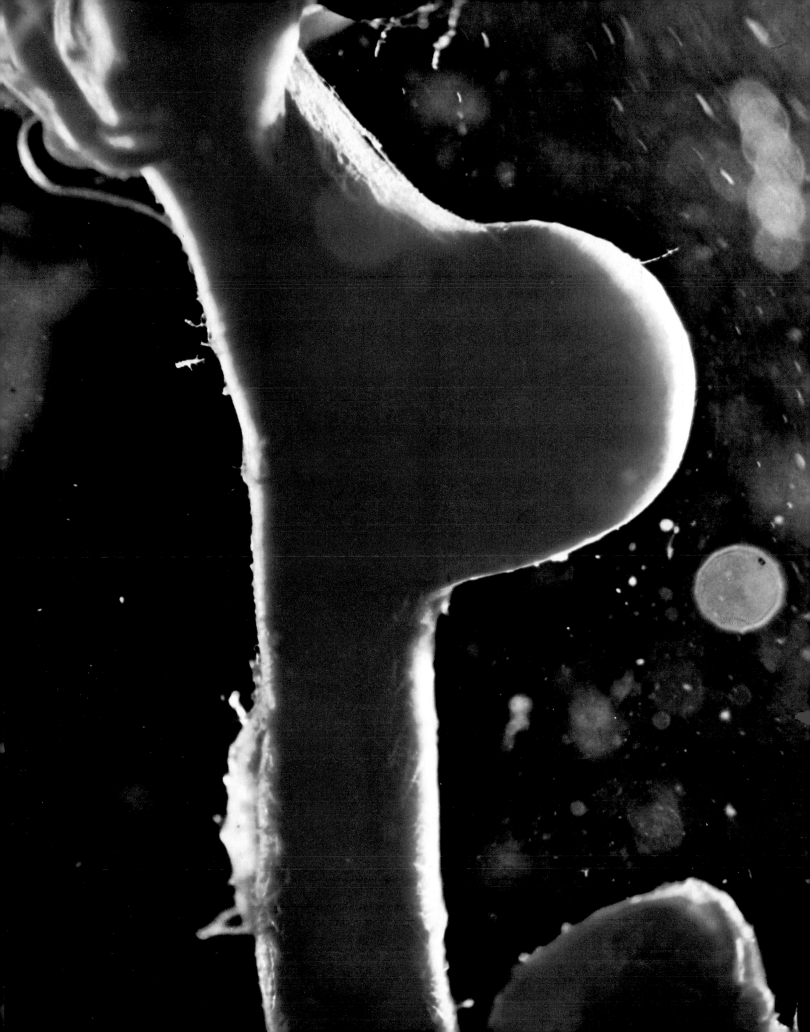

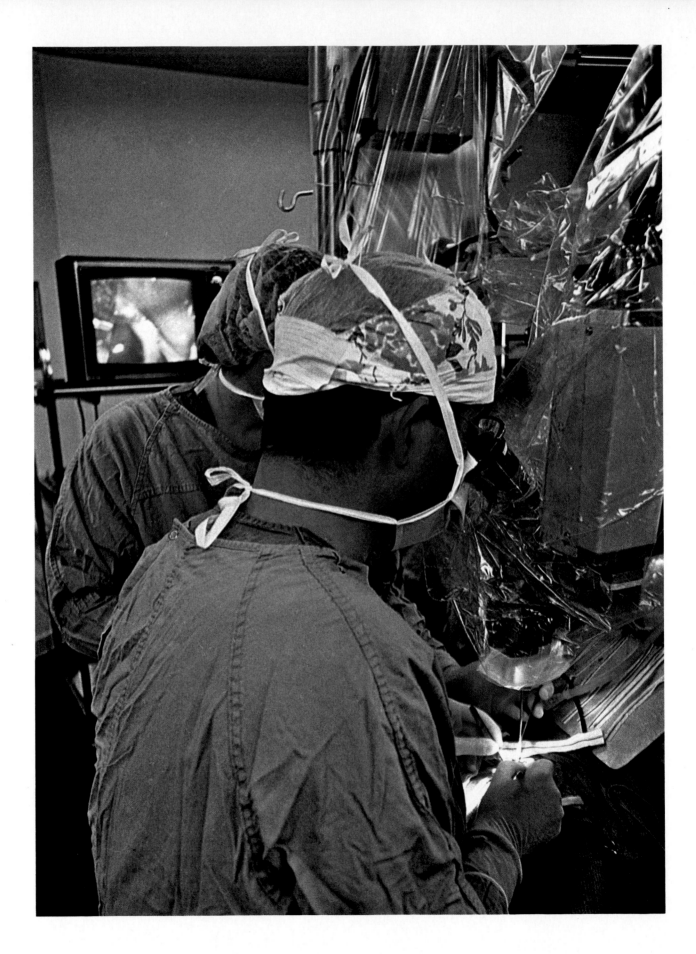

Rerouting blood vessels in the brain, microsurgery cuts to the quick of life. Using fine tools and a microscope, surgeons divert an artery from scalp to brain in hopes of increasing blood supply and preventing stroke.

cannot get through an artery to nourish the brain's cells, serious damage occurs. But if caught in time, an obstruction in the internal carotid artery—a major artery feeding the brain—can be bypassed. Sewing together arteries as thin as pencil lead, neurosurgeons create new channels for blood flow to the brain.

In the hospital, the neurologist first attempts to discover the cause and location of the obstruction in the brain's circulation. Brain damage can be determined by a CAT scan. Radioactive isotope scans, electroencephalograms and spinal fluid examinations can rule out the possibility of other causes, such as a tumor. Next, the patient is injected with special dye, causing the brain's blood vessels to glow on an X-ray angiogram. The blocked artery is indicated by a stoppage of circulating dye. Knowing the size and location of the obstructed artery, doctors will order surgery.

In the operating room, the neurosurgeon feels along the surface of the patient's skull to find an outer scalp artery. This artery must be roughly the same size and nearby the brain artery inside the skull to which it will be attached. Under the microscope, the neurosurgeon makes an incision alongside the scalp artery. After separating it from the surrounding skin, he cuts through the muscle below to the skull. Using the trephine, a miniature cylindrical saw, he cuts a small hole through the skull, exposing the patient's brain. With microscissors he slits, then peels back, the thin, filmy membranes covering the brain. To select which branch of the internal carotid artery will receive the bypass, the neurosurgeon adjusts the microscope to magnify the surface arteries about twenty times their actual size.

To prepare both arteries for the new connection, he first must stop circulation in the scalp artery with noncrushing microclips, and snip it in half. Through the hole he then places two clips on the brain artery. Between the clips, he cuts an oval opening to fit the diagonal end of the scalp artery and eases a Teflon tube inside to keep the artery open.

Increasing the magnification, the neurosurgeon feeds the scalp artery through the skull opening, and sews it to the brain artery with a curved microneedle as fine as a baby's eyelash. With

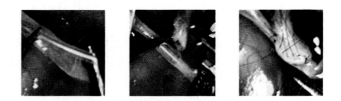

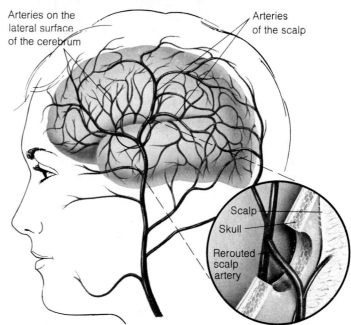

Fitted with a tube to keep its shape, top left, a brain artery receives a scalp (donor) artery, center. The two are sewn together, at right. The new connection will bring more blood to a starving brain. The diagram pinpoints the bypass.

Skulls fused at birth, Elisa and Lisa Hansen underwent a sixteen-hour operation to divide shared cerebral arteries. Delicate microsurgery permitted this, the first such successful parting of Siamese twins.

In critical condition after the operation, the twins two years later, right, suffered few and negligible aftereffects. Doctors say the brain's regenerative power will ensure them normal lives.

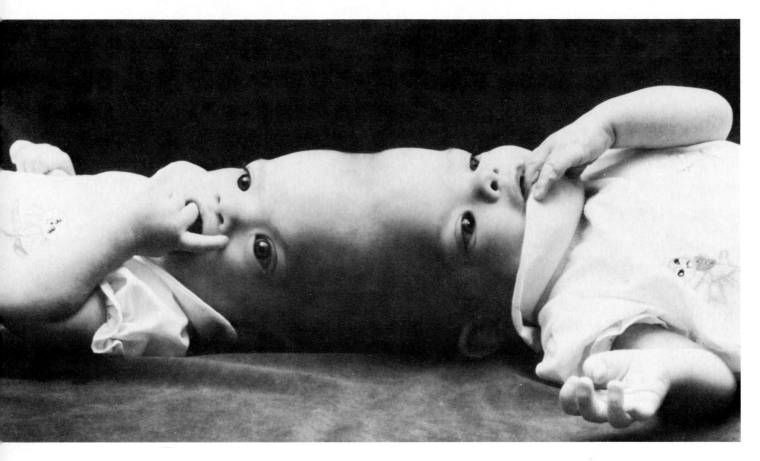

thread four times as slender, he makes about twenty tiny stitches, or microsutures. When he removes the clips, the blood flow immediately returns. A successful bypass can restore from 50 to 100 percent of the brain's blood flow supplied by a healthy internal carotid artery.

Microsurgical techniques have also boosted the success rate for operations to remove aneurysms, or swelling, bubble-shaped weaknesses in the walls of brain arteries. Using minute metal clips, neurosurgeons can cut off aneurysms from the arteries, allowing them to be collapsed by pricking. The clips can be left in without harming the patient. High-powered operating microscopes enable surgeons to remove pituitary tumors through the nose and sew tiny, injured brain nerves back together. Microsurgical advances may soon make nerve transplants possible.

The historic separation of the infants Elisa and Lisa Hansen, Siamese twins joined at the head,

would not have been possible without improved microsurgical instruments. The sixteen-hour operation in 1979 is the first successful separation of twins with total craniopagus, the sharing of blood vessels as well as skulls.

Doctors at the University of Utah Medical Center first performed four preliminary operations in which they tied off the shared blood vessels, a strategy aimed at reducing the chances of hemorrhaging or swelling after actual separation.

During the separation procedure, doctors cut the veins and sealed off bleeding. But then they discovered a potentially disastrous complication: the girls' brains had begun to fuse at the back of their heads. Dividing the brain tissue evenly between each twin, doctors cut the wedge of shared brain matter along natural cleavage lines. When the twins were finally separated, doctors placed a protective covering of treated skin over their exposed brains, then attached flaps of skin from the

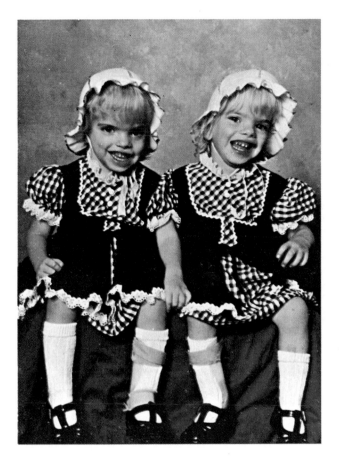

cells containing dopamine from the brains of rat fetuses. The grafts relieved Parkinsonian tremors in many of the rats. In some cases, the transplanted cells even grew. Scientists are especially surprised that none of the rats have shown signs of rejecting the grafts, since other tissue transplants are often rejected by the host body.

Researchers believe brain grafts might relieve Parkinson's disease and other human neurological disorders as well. But finding brain tissue for human grafts would be difficult, since it appears that only fetal or infant brain grafts are effective. "There is a big gap between rats and humans," cautions Richard J. Wyatt, a psychiatrist at the National Institutes of Health.

While the technical, ethical and legal obstacles to human brain grafts and transplants might never be overcome, brain stimulators are already in use. Tiny implanted electrodes connected to computers or portable electronic devices now help relieve chronic pain, control epileptic seizures and restore movement to limbs paralyzed by stroke. More sophisticated devices have been used experimentally to create artificial vision and hearing for the blind and the deaf.

The vision prosthesis entirely bypasses the eye. Placed on the visual cortex of the brain, a Teflon plate containing sixty-four electrodes is connected to a computer through wires which run out through the scalp above the ear. The computer reconstructs an image from a television camera and determines which electrodes to stimulate in order to produce varying patterns of light flashes called phosphenes. Patients see these flashes in the form of Braille letters and simple shapes. The device is not practical, however, since it cannot be taken out of the laboratory.

Dr. William Dobelle, director of the Division of Artificial Organs, Department of Surgery at Columbia University, hopes to construct a portable vision prosthesis using microminiaturized components. He also aims to improve image resolution by implanting a strip containing 256 electrodes into each hemisphere. The resulting pictures, he says, would at best resemble those flashed on an electronic scoreboard at a stadium.

Dobelle's work has been challenged by some scientists who question the safety of direct, con-

girls' legs as an outer layer. Nearly two years after this dangerous and pioneering operation, the twins' only apparent problems are a slight numbness and slowness in moving.

The most radical form of neurosurgery, the brain transplant, has already been performed with surprising success on Rhesus monkeys. At the Brain Research Laboratory in Cleveland's Metropolitan General Hospital, Dr. Robert White has been transplanting monkey brains for the last several years. White believes human brain transplants would be possible once scientists devise a way to make the severed spinal cords between the brain and body grow back together. But he also foresees tremendous ethical obstacles to performing such operations.

Less awesome than the total brain transplant is the grafting of selected areas of the brain. In a recent experiment, rats suffering from a disorder similar to Parkinson's disease received grafts of tinuous brain stimulation. They also doubt that the images produced would really be useful to the blind. Nonetheless, this research on brain stimulation has brought forward important issues of concern to researchers seeking to aid persons with sensory impairment.

Controlling Seizures

Improvements in drug-monitoring tests, drug therapy and diagnostic techniques help 80 percent of all epileptic patients to lead nearly normal lives. The second most common neurological disorder after stroke, epilepsy afflicts two million Americans. Epileptic seizures — sudden abnormal firings of brain cells — can result in attention lapses, hallucinations or convulsions. While head injury, brain disease or alcoholism can lead to epilepsy, often the cause is unknown.

A recently initiated cooperative program involving government and the drug industry has intensified the search for new antiepileptic drugs. Three medications recently introduced in this country have proven both safe and effective. Doctors are not sure how these drugs work, but there is evidence that the newest drug, valproic acid, prevents seizures by increasing the quantity of the neurotransmitter GABA (gamma-aminobutyric acid) in epileptic brain cells.

Doctors now use electronic equipment to study epileptics who suffer intractable seizures. In a special room, television cameras videotape a patient experiencing a seizure, while an EEG machine simultaneously records brain waves. Doctors later correlate the physical manifestations of the seizure with brain-wave patterns. This technique, called intensive monitoring, helps scientists establish standardized clinical definitions for specific types of seizures.

New methods for measuring the level of drugs in the bloodstream have now eliminated what was often lengthy trial and error to determine the proper dosage for each patient. The Enzyme Multiple Immunoassay Technique (EMIT) and gas liquid chromatography (GLC), performed routinely in most laboratories, can immediately determine how a particular drug affects the body. One company soon hopes to introduce a drug-monitoring system for use in doctors' offices.

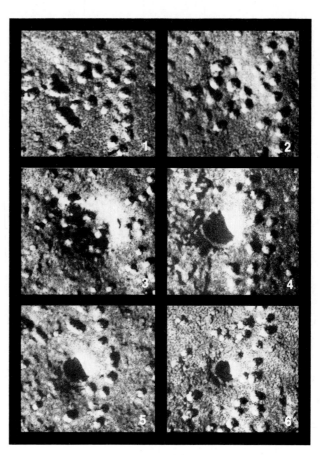

Viewed from across the synapse, the transmitting end of the terminal button is magnified half a million times. In this freeze-slamming sequence, taken in a quarter of a second, the vesicle containing neurotransmitter chemicals reaches the surface of the button (1 and 2), blows open and spills its chemicals into the gap (3 and 4) and then begins to close (5 and 6). With freeze slamming, the rapid freezing and fracture of tissue, scientists hope to find clues to such diseases as epilepsy and multiple sclerosis.

The mind itself may play a role in curing disease. In 1964, Norman Cousins, editor of *Saturday Review* magazine, was stricken with a degenerative disease of connective tissue. Doctors said his chances of surviving the illness were one in five hundred. But, spurred on by the book *The Stress of Life*, Cousins decided to fight the odds. Author Hans Selye showed that negative emotions can upset body chemistry and bring on disease. Could positive emotions have the opposite effect, Cousins wondered? He set out on a "systematic pursuit of the salutary emotions," watching Marx Brothers' movies and "Candid Camera" television shows to alleviate chronic pain. Incredibly, almost every symptom disappeared.

Perhaps most remarkable of all, there is growing evidence that the brain and other parts of the central nervous system can adapt to trauma and even heal themselves. Traditional scientific belief has long held that alcoholism can cause permanent brain damage. But CAT scans of recovered alcoholics reveal that some brain cells had actually regenerated. In some patients, cell repair was evident after just three weeks of abstinence.

Scientists are looking to the future when they can rebuild severed spinal cords, and thereby reduce the paralysis that follows. At Georgetown University in Washington, D.C., neurosurgeon Carl C. Kao has succeeded in implanting healthy nerve tissue onto the severed spinal cords of dogs. The grafts formed a healing bridge across the tear, enabling the dogs to walk.

As scientists penetrate the substance of the brain with grafts and transplants, pacemaker machines and drugs for controlling brain functions, a fundamental question arises: To what extent can we manipulate the brain — precious sustainer of life, physical basis of mind and soul — before the very essence of life itself is transformed?

The challenge of unfolding the brain's mysteries is a compelling one. To neuroscientist Francis O. Schmitt, "Whether one likes it or not, man has embarked on the greatest of human experiments . . . that of determining whether . . . man can discover the mechanism of thinking, and whether, by so doing, he can achieve new orders of understanding . . . the dimensions of his own nature."

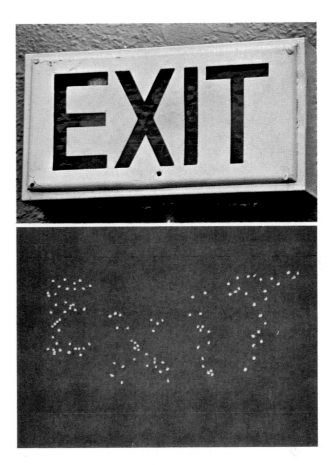

A simple EXIT sign, above, taken for granted by the sighted, would read like a neon miracle to a blind person with electrodes implanted on the visual centers of his brain. Perception transforms the points of light, called phosphenes, into the letters' rough configuration, below. In the future, vision prostheses could offer the sightless a glimpse of the world outside the laboratory.

Glossary

activation-synthesis theory an explanation of dreaming holding that dreams are attempts by the cerebral cortex to impose meaning on random neuron firings in the brain during REM periods.

afferent a term meaning directed inward toward a center. Afferent nerve impulses travel from muscles and glands into the central nervous system.

amino acids organic molecules that join together to form proteins.

amygdala an almond-shaped mass of nerves situated at the front of the limbic system; thought to play an important role in feelings of rage and aggression.

aneurysm a bubblelike swelling in the wall of an artery which may enlarge, pressing against body organs, or burst. An aneurysm in the brain can lead to stroke.

angiogram an X-ray picture of blood vessels, which can reveal brain disorders such as strokes, blood clots and tumors.

aphasia a language impairment resulting from brain damage. The various forms of aphasia involve an inability to either comprehend or produce written or spoken language.

association cortex a portion of the cerebral cortex which has no direct connections with other parts of the central nervous system. It is thought to integrate sensory and motor information and to account, in large part, for man's higher intelligence.

association fibers the most numerous of three categories of white matter within the brain; nerve fibers which link together all regions of the cortex within the same cerebral hemisphere.

auditory cortex a region of the cerebral cortex, lying mostly within the temporal lobes, where sounds are received.

autonomic nervous system the division of the central nervous system that regulates such involuntary processes as breathing, heart rate and digestion. Its two subdivisions, the sympathetic and parasympathetic systems, have opposite functions. The hypothalamus ensures that they work in harmony, adjusting their activities to changing bodily needs.

axon a long fiber extending from the cell body of a neuron which conveys impulses to neighboring neurons.

basal ganglia four clusters of neurons at the base of the brain which help regulate body movements. Its components are the amygdala, putamen, globus pallidus and caudate nucleus.

behaviorism a school of psychology which studies only those aspects of behavior that are objectively observable.

beta-endorphin an opiatelike peptide containing thirty-one amino acids, found in the pituitary gland.

biofeedback the technique in which electronic equipment is used to teach subjects how to regulate physical processes normally thought beyond conscious control.

blood-brain barrier a protective system which prevents certain toxic chemicals and other substances in the bloodstream from entering the brain. It is believed to consist of the walls of capillaries and glial membranes.

brainstem the range of bulges that forms the central core of the brain, running from the top of the spinal cord into the middle of the brain.

Broca's area the region within the left frontal lobe that controls the flow of words from brain to mouth.

cell body the main portion of a neuron, containing the nucleus.

central nervous system the part of the nervous system consisting of the brain and spinal cord.

cerebellum the twin-lobed, oval structure behind the brainstem responsible for coordinating movements.

cerebral cortex the thin, convoluted outer layer of the cerebral hemispheres, rich in nerve cells, and the birthplace of man's higher mental functions.

cerebrospinal fluid the transparent liquid found in the ventricles of the brain and in the spaces surrounding the brain and spinal cord. It helps protect the brain by cushioning it against blows.

cerebrum the largest portion of the brain, consisting of left and right cerebral hemispheres.

circadian rhythm an internal time-keeping mechanism, based roughly on a twenty-four-hour cycle, which governs many bodily systems.

commissural fibers nerve fibers that link together both cerebral hemispheres; one of three types of white matter.

computerized axial tomography (CAT) a technique for diagnosing brain disorders. As an X-ray beam passes through a thin section of the head, detectors record how much radiation the slice absorbed, then relay the information to a computer. The computer mathematically reconstructs the data and projects an image onto a video screen.

corpus callosum the bridge of nerve fibers connecting the left and right cerebral hemispheres; it permits the exchange of information between them.

deep structure the underlying meaning of a sentence which, according to psycholinguistic theory, is innately understood.

dendrite a short, fine branch extending from the cell body of a neuron which receives impulses through synaptic contacts with nearby neurons.

dopamine a neurotransmitter found in high concentrations in the basal ganglia region of the brain; dopamine excess or deficiency is thought to contribute to severe mental illness.

dorsal pertaining to the back surface of an object.

Dynamic Spatial Reconstructor (DSR) a machine that produces three-dimensional, stop-action images of the body's interior. A battery of X-ray guns sends pictures to a computer, which then reassembles the image electronically.

efferent a term meaning conducted outward from a center. Efferent nerve impulses arise from within the central nervous system and travel outward.

electrical stimulation of the brain (ESB) the application of a mild electrical current to electrodes implanted in the brain; used to map brain functions and study behavior.

electrode a solid conductor used either for sending electrical current into specific brain regions, or for recording the brain's electrical activity.

electroencephalograph (EEG) a machine that records electrical activity of the brain, from electrodes attached to the scalp. The EEG shows fluctuations in the amplitude and frequency of brain waves.

endocrine glands organs which secrete hormones directly into the bloodstream or the lymphatic fluid. Included are the thyroid, pancreas, pituitary and adrenal glands.

endoneurium a network of connective tissue woven throughout each peripheral nerve, separating and linking individual nerve fibers.

endorphins a term used generally to refer to all substances in the body having opiatelike qualities, including enkephalins and beta-endorphin.

engram a permanent memory trace in the brain; the hypothetical alteration of brain tissue resulting from a psychical experience.

enkephalins two brain peptides, each containing five amino acids, which interact with opiate receptors to relieve pain.

enzymes proteins, produced by cells, which speed up biochemical reactions.

epilepsy a neurological disability marked by the sudden, abnormal discharge of brain cells, causing convulsions, hallucinations, loss of consciousness or attention lapse.

epineurium a dense sheath of connective tissue which envelops each peripheral nerve.

equipotentiality a theory maintaining the equal distribution of memory and other mental processes throughout functional units of the cortex.

evoked potentials minute changes in the electrical activity of specific brain regions during repeated presentations of a stimulus or the performance of a specific task. Recorded by scalp electrodes, these brain waves are identified by a computer and can reveal a variety of brain disorders.

fascicles bundles of nerve fibers; subdivisions of the connective tissue sheath (epineurium) surrounding peripheral nerves.

frontal lobe one of four regions of the cerebral cortex. The frontal lobe lies directly behind the forehead. The hindmost part of this lobe contains the motor cortex, but the function of the remaining portion is unclear. Some researchers theorize that foresight, planning and personality are located here.

glia "nerve glue"; special cells that surround each neuron, providing support and nourishment.

glucose a simple sugar converted from carbohydrates during digestion; the chief source of fuel for brain cells.

gray matter tissue in the brain and spinal cord consisting of the cell bodies of neurons. In the brain, gray matter is located on the surface; the gray matter of the spinal cord is interior.

habituation the process by which the brain gradually adapts to a novel sensation and no longer notices it; regulated by the reticular formation.

hippocampus a U-shaped formation in the limbic system, thought to play an important role in learning and short-term memory.

holography a photographic technique in which a three-dimensional image is produced from interference patterns created by a split laser beam.

Holography has been proposed as a model for memory and perceptual processes.

hormones chemical substances produced by endocrine glands which stimulate the activity of certain organs.

humanistic psychology a school of psychology that emphasizes the uniqueness of human beings and their potential for self-fulfillment; it holds that each person is responsible for his own actions.

hypothalamus a small neuron cluster at the base of the forebrain, essential in coordinating central nervous system functions, including the regulation of body temperature, sex drive, thirst and hunger. It also controls endocrine activity and plays an important role in emotions of pain and pleasure.

interference theory the belief that forgetting occurs when memories interfere with each other, i.e., when an old memory blocks out new information, or vice versa.

language universals in psycholinguistics, the hypothesis of basic linguistic uniformities through which children acquire language.

limbic system a group of structures at the base of the forebrain involved in emotions and behavior.

medulla oblongata part of the brainstem linking the spinal cord below with the pons above; controls respiration and blood circulation.

metabolism the sum of all chemical and physical reactions in the body necessary for maintaining life; in particular, the conversion of food substances into energy.

microelectrode extremely slender glass or metal electrodes which are inserted into individual brain cells to record electrical activity.

microsurgery surgery using high-powered microscopes for greater precision. This technique has broadened the scope of neurosurgery, making commonplace brain operations that were once believed impossible.

morpheme the smallest meaningful unit of language, e.g., a suffix, prefix or single-syllable word.

multiple sclerosis a degenerative disease of the nervous system in which the myelin sheath surrounding nerve fibers is destroyed, then replaced by scar tissue. The disease can lead to partial paralysis, blindness, speech disorders and other impairments.

myelin a fatty white substance that covers and insulates each axon.

neuron the basic conducting unit of the nervous system (also called a nerve cell), consisting of a cell body and threadlike projections that conduct electrical impulses. The axon, a single long fiber, transmits the impulses, while shorter extensions called dendrites receive them.

neurotransmitter a chemical; one of approximately thirty messenger molecules that transmit impulses from neuron to neuron. Stored in axon terminals, this chemical substance is released into the synaptic gap when a neuron fires, and locks onto a receiving cell's dendrites.

NREM sleep a series of gradually deepening sleep stages marked by a decline in brain activity and body processes.

nuclear magnetic resonance (NMR) a scanning technique used to diagnose tumors and other abnormalities. When exposed to a high energy beam, hydrogen atoms within a magnetic field produce electrical signals. Processed by a computer, these signals yield a color cross section showing hydrogen density of body tissue and structures.

nucleolus the small, spherical structure within the nucleus of a cell, containing RNA and protein.

occipital lobe the lower portion of the cerebral cortex, containing the visual cortex.

parietal lobe a region of the cerebral cortex located between the frontal and occipital lobes; the receiving area for touch sensations and information about spatial orientation.

Parkinson's disease a progressive neurological disorder marked by tremors of the face and hands, muscular rigidity, peculiar gait and a masklike facial expression. The disease is thought to be caused by cell degeneration in the basal ganglia region.

peptide a short chain of amino acids.

phonemes basic sounds; the smallest units of speech in any language. Each language has a specific number, e.g., English having forty-five.

pineal gland a cone-shaped organ at the base of the brain whose function in humans is unknown. In some lower animals, it detects light and may influence internal rhythms.

pituitary gland the body's "master gland," situated below its controlling organ, the hypothalamus. This gland secretes hormones which regulate other endocrine glands, controlling growth, reproduction and numerous metabolic processes.

"pleasure centers" nerve circuits within the hypothalamus and other limbic system sites where pleasurable feelings are thought to originate.

pons a band of nerve fibers at the front of the brainstem bridging the left and right halves of the cerebellum.

positron-emission transaxial tomography (PETT) a tool which produces images of body metabolism used to diagnose brain functions and disorders. The PETT scanner traces radiation through body tissue, following the injection of a radioactive isotope. Analyzing information recorded by the scanner, a computer transforms the data into a color video image of the body's biochemistry.

prefrontal lobe part of the frontal lobe lying directly behind the forehead. Its function may be related to the ability to plan and to make choices.

projection fibers one of three types of white matter, they convey impulses between the cerebral cortex and other parts of the nervous system.

protein a molecule present in every cell, made up of a sequence of amino acids. Proteins are essential in building and repairing body tissue.

protoplasm a translucent, jellylike substance within and surrounding a cell; the essential living matter of cells.

psychoanalysis the therapeutic technique developed by Freud in which buried emotional conflicts are brought into conscious awareness through free association and dream interpretation.

Purkinje cells a layer of large, flask-shaped nerve cells in the cortex of the cerebellum. Each Purkinje cell has numerous dendrites which may make up to 100,000 synaptic links with other nerve fibers.

pyramidal cells large, triangular cells found in the motor areas of the cortex. Also known as Betz cells, these neurons activate muscular movements, each neuron governing a specific part of a muscle.

radioisotope scanning a diagnostic method that detects and records radiation levels in specific organs. Once a patient has been injected with a radioactive isotope, an electronic device then converts this information into picture form.

receptors specialized cells located in sense organs, skin, muscles and joints. They convert information into nerve impulses, then transmit the impulses to sensory neurons.

reflex arc a nerve circuit used for involuntary, rapid response. Messages travel from receptors to sensory neurons, then to motor neurons in the spinal cord which direct the appropriate response.

"relaxation response" the combined physiological changes, including reductions in blood pressure, heart rate and oxygen consumption, brought about through certain techniques of meditation.

REM sleep the stage of sleep in which vivid dreaming occurs. REM is the acronym for "rapid eye movements," one of the distinguishing physical signs of this sleep period.

reticular formation a dense web of neurons in the brainstem that regulates consciousness and channels the brain's attention. The reticular formation and its pathways running from the spinal cord to the cortex are known as the reticular activating system (RAS).

ribonucleic acid (RNA) a large molecule found in all living cells. RNA transmits genetic information and synthesizes proteins.

sensory register a step in recording memory. The register holds information briefly after it enters the brain. Most of its contents are lost after a second or two; the rest filters through to short-term memory banks.

septum pellucidum a thin, triangular membrane in the brain connected to the hypothalamus; believed to contain nerve centers for pleasure.

Skinner box a box equipped with various instruments, used by experimental psychologists to study how laboratory animals learn; named after its developer, behavioral psychologist B. F. Skinner.

sociobiology the study of the genetic basis of social behavior.

spinal cord the portion of the nervous system enclosed by the bones of the spinal column; it extends from the base of the brainstem to the second lumbar vertebra. The spinal cord is the body's main nerve circuit, carrying out reflex actions and sending nerve impulses to and from the brain through its ascending and descending nerve tracts.

stroke a sudden interruption in blood supply to the brain, caused either by

hemorrhage of a blood vessel or blockage in a vein or artery supplying the brain. Death or permanent damage, including paralysis, blindness or speech impairment, may result.

synapse the microscopic gap between two adjacent nerve cells. Chemical neurotransmitters carry nerve impulses across the synapse.

synaptic vesicle one of numerous tiny pouches contained within the terminal button at the end of an axon. When the vesicle erupts, it spills a chemical transmitter substance into the synapse.

syntax grammar; a set of rules for arranging words into phrases and sentences in a given language.

temporal lobe the area of the cerebral cortex located near the temples of the skull that contains centers for hearing and memory.

thalamus a twin-lobed mass of nerve cells at the top of the brainstem containing relay centers for sensory and motor information to and from the brain.

triune brain an evolutionary model of the brain as a three-layered structure. Each layer represents a different evolutionary stage. The oldest layer, the reptilian brain, governs vital body functions. The old mammalian brain, the middle layer, is the center for instinct and feeling, and maintains the body's internal equilibrium. The third and latest layer to evolve is the new mammalian brain, or cerebrum, where higher thought processes arise.

ultradian rhythm the continuous ninety-minute cycle of fast and slow brain waves which produces alternating periods of mental excitement and calm.

unconscious the Freudian term for the portion of the psyche not subject to direct observation; it contains repressed desires and instincts.

ventral pertaining to the front surface of an object.

ventricles four interconnected cavities within the brain which contain cerebrospinal fluid. These hollows are expansions of the central canal of the spinal cord.

visual cortex the part of the occipital lobe at the back of the cerebrum. It receives and interprets what the eye sees.

Wernicke's area part of the left temporal lobe where language is perceived.

white matter parts of the brain and spinal cord composed mostly of whitish nerve fibers (axons) and no nerve cell bodies.

Photographic Credits

Title
2, Howard Sochurek/Woodfin Camp & Associates.

Introduction
6, C.P. Hodge, Montreal Neurological Institute

The Divinest Part
8, Photo Bibliothèque Nationale, Paris. 10, Zentralbibliothek Zürich. 11, National Library of Medicine. 12–13, Royal Library, Windsor Castle; reproduced by gracious permission of Her Majesty Queen Elizabeth II. 14–16, National Library of Medicine. 17, The Bettmann Archive. 18, (top) Culver Pictures (bottom) The Bettmann Archive. 19, The Bettmann Archive. 22, The Bettmann Archive. 23, (top) National Library of Medicine (bottom) Dr. N. A. Lassen.

Landscapes of the Brain
24, Manfred Kage/Peter Arnold, Inc. 28, Manfred Kage/Peter Arnold, Inc. 29, T.A. Woolsey, from DREAMSTAGE © 1977 J.A. Hobson and Hoffmann-La Roche, Inc.

The Electrochemical Brain
36, Manfred Kage/Peter Arnold, Inc. 40, Lennart Nilsson, *Behold Man* (Boston: Little, Brown and Company, 1974). 43, Barbara F. Reese, Marine Biological Laboratory, Woods Hole, Massachusetts. 46, Emmett N. Leith and Juris Upatnieks, "Photography by Laser," *Scientific American*, volume 212, number 6 (June 1965). 48, The Granger Collection, New York. 49, Howard Sochurek/Woodfin Camp & Associates. 50, Miles Herkenham and Candace Pert.

The Gift of Language
52, The Bettmann Archive. 57, Ed Lettau/FPG. 58, Bruno Barbey/Magnum. 59, Henri Cartier-Bresson/Magnum. 63, Paul Fusco/Magnum. 64, Ann Hagen Griffiths, Omni-Photo Communications, Inc. 65, Dan McCoy/Rainbow.

Intelligence and Creativity
66, Brown Brothers. 68, (top) Joe Di Dio/National Education Association (bottom) Erich Hartmann/Magnum. 69, R.L. Thorndike and E.P. Hagen, *Cognitive Abilities Test* © 1972 by permission of The Riverside Publishing Company. 70, (top) Ed Lettau/Photo Researchers (bottom) Margot Granusas/Photo Researchers. 71, (top) Harbutt/Magnum. (bottom) Jen and Des Bartlett/Bruce Coleman, Inc. 74, (left) Picture Collection, Branch Libraries, The New York Public Library (right) Phoenix Art Museum, gift of Mr. and Mrs. Henry R. Luce. 75, Philadelphia Museum of Art, the Louise and Walter Arensberg Collection. 76, (left) © 1969 Rollie McKenna (middle) Henri Dauman/Magnum (right) The Granger Collection, New York. 77, (left) California Institute of Technology (middle & right) The Bettmann Archive. 78, (left) Museum of African Art, Smithsonian Institution, gift of Mrs. Joanne F. duPont (right) Kunstsammlung Nordrhein-Westfalen, Düsseldorf. 79, Collection of Mr. and Mrs. S.I. Newhouse, Jr.

Remembrance of Things Past
80, Collection of Mrs. Robert B. Mayer, Chicago. 86, *Soviet Life Magazine*. 87, Suzanne Szasz. 88–89, Paintings by Sybil, courtesy of Dr. Wilbur.

The Feeling Brain
90, The Bettmann Archive. 92, Dr. Robert B. Livingston, M.D., Professor of Neurosciences, University of California, San Diego. 94–95, Dan McCoy/Rainbow. 97, James Olds, "Pleasure Centers in the Brain," *Scientific American*, volume 195, number 10 (October 1956). 98, Dennis Yeandle/Black Star. 101, Dr. José M.R. Delgado, "Evolution of Physical Control of the Brain," James Arthur Lecture, American Museum of Natural History, New York, 1965. 102, C. Keith Conners, Ph.D., Childrens Hospital National Medical Center. 105, Arthur P. Arnold, UCLA.

Mazes of the Mind
106, Collection Haags Gemeentemuseum © 1981 BEELDRECHT Amsterdam /VAGA, New York. 109, (top & bottom) The Bettmann Archive. 112, Victoria and Albert Museum, Crown Copyright. 113 Cesare Ripa, *Baroque and Rococo Pictorial Imagery* (New York: Dover Publications, Inc., 1971). 114, R. Epstein and R.P. Lanza. 117, Paul Fusco/Magnum. 119, Al Vercoutere, Malibu, California.

Realms of Consciousness
120, Marc Chagall, *Le Visage Bleu* (The Blue Face) © 1981 ADAGP, Paris. 122, Diana Digiacomo/Focus on Sports. 126, (1–3) Reproduced from *Some Must Watch While Some Must Sleep: Exploring the World of Sleep*, by William C. Dement, by permission of W.W. Norton & Company, Inc. © 1972, 1974, 1976 William C. Dement (4) Ernst Niedermeyer, M.D., Johns Hopkins Hospital, Baltimore, Maryland. 127, Christopher Springmann, courtesy of Stephen C. Coburn. 128, Photos © Ted Spagna, courtesy of J.A. Hobson and Hoffmann-La Roche, Inc.; graphs from DREAMSTAGE © 1977 J.A. Hobson and Hoffmann-La Roche, Inc. 130 © Ted Spagna. 131, DREAMSTAGE © 1977 J.A. Hobson and Hoffmann-La Roche, Inc. 132–133, Collection of Ronald K. Siegel. 134, Jonathan T. Wright/Bruce Coleman, Inc. 135, © David Attie.

The Unfolding Tapestry
136, Howard Sochurek/Woodfin Camp & Associates. 139, (top) Dan McCoy /Rainbow (bottom) © 1979 John Ficara /Newsweek. 140 (top) Courtesy of Dr. M.M. Ter-Pogossian, The Edward Mallinckrodt Institute of Radiology, St. Louis, Missouri. 140–141, Dan McCoy /Rainbow. 142–143, Brookhaven National Laboratory and New York University Medical Center. 145, Lennart Nilsson. 146–147, Dan McCoy/Rainbow. 148, University of Utah Medical Illustration. 149, Attorney Darrell G. Renstrom. 150, National Institutes of Health. 151, (top) Donald Dietz/Stock Boston, (bottom) Created by biomedical engineer and technical journalist Albert F. Shackil, based on his article in *IEEE Spectrum*, September, 1980.

Index

Page numbers in bold type indicate location of illustrations.